The Physician as Patient

A Clinical Handbook for
Mental Health Professionals

The Physician as Patient

A Clinical Handbook for Mental Health Professionals

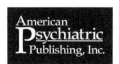

Michael F. Myers, M.D.

Director, Marital Therapy Clinic, St. Paul's Hospital;
Clinical Professor, Department of Psychiatry
University of British Columbia
Vancouver, Canada

Glen O. Gabbard, M.D.

Brown Foundation Chair of
Psychoanalysis and Professor
Department of Psychiatry and Behavioral Sciences;
Director, Baylor Psychiatry Clinic
Baylor College of Medicine;
Training and Supervising Analyst
Houston–Galveston Psychoanalytic Institute
Houston, Texas

American **Psychiatric** Publishing, Inc.

Washington, DC
London, England

Copyright © 2008 American Psychiatric Publishing, Inc.
ALL RIGHTS RESERVED

The first-person account in Chapter 11 is reprinted from Myers MF, Fine C: *Touched by Suicide: Hope and Healing After Loss.* New York, Gotham/Penguin Books, 2006. Used with permission of the Penguin Group.

Manufactured in the United States of America on acid-free paper
11   10   09   08   07   5   4   3   2   1
First Edition

Typeset in Adobe's Akzidenz Grotesk and Minion.

American Psychiatric Publishing, Inc.
1000 Wilson Boulevard, Arlington, VA 22209-3901
www.appi.org

Library of Congress Cataloging-in-Publication Data
Myers, Michael F.
   The physician as patient : a clinical handbook for mental health professionals / Michael F. Myers, Glen O. Gabbard. — 1st ed.
      p. ; cm.
   Includes bibliographical references and index.
   ISBN 978-1-58562-312-9 (pbk. : alk. paper) 1. Physicians—Mental health.
2. Physicians—Psychology. I. Gabbard, Glen O. II. Title. [DNLM: 1. Mental Disorders. 2. Physicians—psychology. 3. Psychotherapy—methods. WM 140 M996p 2008]
   RC451.4.P5M94 2008
   616.89′14—dc22   2007041796

British Library Cataloguing in Publication Data
A CIP record is available from the British Library.

Contents

Introduction

What happens when physicians become ill? How easy or difficult is it for physicians to relinquish the role of caretaker and to be cared for by others? What is unique about the psychological makeup of physicians, as well as the culture of medicine, that facilitates or impedes timely and comprehensive diagnosis and treatment? When doctors behave badly or out of character at work, what factors underlie such behavior, and what can be done about it? In assessing and treating physicians, what strategies are useful to assure accuracy while simultaneously diminishing morbidity and relieving suffering? And given the frightening rate of suicide in physicians, how can we—a collective of individuals who care about doctors—lower the number of lives lost each year?

The foregoing questions are a smattering of those we attempt to answer in this volume. We both have been working in the field of physician health throughout our careers. Curiosity about the women and men who become physicians, especially their strengths and vulnerabilities, has sparked and informed our research, clinical insights, teaching, scholarly activity, and advocacy near and far.

Michael Myers first became interested in the problems of physicians when he was a medical student. Tragically, one of his roommates, another medical student, killed himself. The silence was deafening as everyone buried themselves in their studies. Later, when Dr. Myers was a resident in psychiatry, he gained some initial experience treating physicians (and their spouses and children) under supervision. This gave him a nascent comfort level treating colleagues as he grew into becoming a "doctors' doctor" after his residency. This resulted, in 1988, in *Doctors' Marriages: A Look at the Problems and Their Solutions* (now in its second edition; Myers 1994). For many years, Dr. Myers has served on the Committee on Physician Health, Illness, and Impairment of the American Psychiatric Association, and in 2001 he founded the Section on Physician Health of the Canadian Psychiatric Association. He continues to teach half-time at the University of British Columbia and to see private patients, all of whom are medical students, physicians, and their families.

Glen Gabbard began his pursuit of knowledge about physician health as a young psychiatrist at the Menninger Clinic. Along with Dr. Roy Menninger, he led continuing education workshops for physicians and their families each summer in Colorado. Physicians and their spouses attended from across the country. They were neither impaired nor in trouble, yet they all recited similar narratives about the struggles balancing work and family when one or both spouses had a medical career. These workshops culminated in *Medical Marriages* (Gabbard and Menninger 1988). Several years later, Dr. Gabbard, during his term as director of the Menninger Hospital, founded the Professionals in Crisis Unit to provide specialized treatment for physicians and others in distress. In his role as director of the Baylor Psychiatry Clinic, he now continues on a weekly basis to evaluate physicians for licensing boards, physician health organizations, and hospital risk-management committees.

This volume is an amalgam of our combined perspectives and experiences in understanding and treating a cohort of human beings who are frequently misunderstood and inadequately treated. Our particular areas of knowledge and expertise usefully complement each other. However, we both contributed to all chapters in the book, resulting in two voices instead of one throughout.

We have divided the book into three parts. The first, "Physician Characteristics and Vulnerabilities," comprises three chapters. Chapter 1 forms the bedrock of much of what follows. In this chapter, we outline the most common personality characteristics of doctors and how physicians are shaped by the values, expectations, and responsibilities of the profession itself. Resilience and susceptibility to stress and illness are key concepts. In Chapter 2 we highlight the diversity of the world of medicine by describing some of the unique features of and challenges for physicians who are members of minority groups, including International Medical Graduates, who form a significant portion of the physician workforce in North America. Chapter 3 addresses a most important charge for medical institutions, licensing authorities, and physicians themselves—physician evaluation. This important chapter is intentionally prescriptive and far-ranging, encompassing the many clinical, humanistic, ethical, and often legal dimensions of the evaluative process.

Part II, "Diagnostic and Treatment Issues in the Distressed and Distressing Physician," contains four chapters. In this section, we describe the most common medical and psychiatric illnesses in physicians (including addictions). We also address the disruptive physician and physicians with personality disorders as well as the complex and increasingly important subject of boundary violations among physicians. Our objective here is to outline key diagnostic and treatment imperatives to make certain that physicians with these illnesses or problem behaviors receive thorough and clinically sophisticated attention—both for their own sake and for the sake of others.

The third and final part is called "Prevention, General Treatment Principles, and Rehabilitation." As the title suggests, we cover many aspects of primary, secondary, and tertiary prevention in the five chapters included here. Our perspective is always biopsychosocial as we advocate integrated care for all physicians. Having outlined many psychopharmacological treatment strategies in Part II, we focus more intensely on psychotherapy here. Three of the more common modalities—psychodynamic, cognitive-behavioral, and couples therapies—are described in detail because so many physician-patients require and respond favorably to these forms of therapy. Also covered in depth is physician suicide—assessment and treatment of the suicidal physician and the aftermath of physician suicide. We hope that we shine some light on a dark, stigmatized, and too long ignored reality for some physicians and their families.

This book is designed for the many people who seek to understand physicians. The readership includes, but is not limited to, clinicians—psychiatrists, primary care and consultant physicians, addiction medicine specialists, and mental health professionals such as psychologists, clinical social workers, and psychiatric nurses who treat physicians and their families. Its reach extends as well to licensing board professionals, physician health organizations, hospital risk-management committees, medical administrators, medical school deans of undergraduate and postgraduate education, and residency program directors.

Throughout this work we have included many case examples to illustrate important observations and key principles. To preserve confidentiality and privacy, all of the stories are heavily disguised or are composites of many patients from our private practices or those of colleagues.

We wish to thank Dr. Robert Hales, Editor-in-Chief, and John McDuffie, Editorial Director, of American Psychiatric Publishing, Inc., for inviting us to write this book. They had the wisdom to perceive a need for such a resource, and their editorial vision has helped us with its form and structure. We are grateful to Greg Kuny, Managing Editor, for helping to shape the book into its final form. Drs. Mike Gendel and Joyce Davidson graciously read chapters and offered helpful feedback. Diane Trees Clay tirelessly worked on the manuscript and references and was indispensable. Finally, we want to thank all of our patients, who are also our colleagues. They have taught us much about ourselves and have entrusted us with their care. It is a privilege to work with them.

Michael F. Myers, M.D.
Glen O. Gabbard, M.D.

PART I

PHYSICIAN CHARACTERISTICS AND VULNERABILITIES

The Psychology of Physicians and the Culture of Medicine

Dr. Jonathan Drummond-Webb was a rising star in the field of pediatric heart surgery. Born in Johannesburg, South Africa, he came to the United States in 1995 to do a surgical fellowship. In 1997 he did a second fellowship at the prestigious Cleveland Clinic. While there, he became the surgical director of pediatric cardiac and lung transplantation. Finally, in 2001 he was named chief of pediatric and congenital cardiac surgery at the Arkansas Children's Hospital in Little Rock, Arkansas. There he was the first endowed chair in pediatric and congenital cardiac surgery. Three years after arriving, on the day after Christmas, he killed himself.

In the midst of the shock and grief, Dr. Jonathan R. Bates, President and Chief Executive Officer of Arkansas Children's Hospital, made the following observation: "Some would say they saved 98 out of 100; he looked at it and said, 'I lost two out of 100'" (Associated Press 2004).

Dr. Drummond-Webb's case is on the extreme end of a continuum. Most physicians do not end up killing themselves. Even though the act of suicide is a complex phenomenon involving some convergence of genes, psychology, and psychosocial stressors, we can often learn something fundamental about the psychology of physicians by studying the lives of those with the most tragic outcomes. The term "impaired physician" can lead us to a form of binary thinking in which a physician either "is" or "is not" impaired. Clinical experience with physician-patients suggests that impairment occurs on a continuum. Certain stressors inherent in the culture of medicine interact with preexisting psychological characteristics of those who enter medicine to pose certain occupational hazards to virtually all physicians. The most sensible preventive approach is to recognize the vulnerabilities and stressors inherent in the practice of medicine and take measures to diminish, eradicate, or at least manage them efficiently.

Dr. Bates's observations about Dr. Drummond-Webb, for example, resonate with most physicians to some degree. He painted a portrait of a man who was haunted by his failures. His many successful accomplishments somehow did not compensate for his occasional unsuccessful attempts to save a child in distress. We do not, of course, know all of the factors that contributed to Dr. Drummond-Webb's suicide. He may have suffered from personal strains or unrecognized depression. Nevertheless, the perfectionism and self-recrimination Dr. Bates describes in Dr. Drummond-Webb are traits common to most physicians and can be a source of torment even for those who do not become suicidal.

What Kind of Person Enters Medicine?

Any consideration of the psychological profile of people who enter medical school must begin with a recognition that medical students represent a range of personality types. We may see some who are shy and avoidant of social relatedness. Others may be arrogant and narcissistic as a way of dealing with their insecurity. Still others may be histrionic and attention seeking. A few may even have antisocial features that lead to corrupt practices later in their careers. However, despite all these variations, a number of core features are found in the majority of physicians, largely because it is difficult to succeed without these psychological characteristics. Perfectionism, for example, is a common theme among medical students and graduate physicians. One might argue that the kind of conscientiousness associated with perfectionism is even necessary to get into medical school and to succeed once there. Hence the perfectionism that may have contributed to Dr. Drummond-Webb's suicide is not entirely unfamiliar to students who never contemplate suicide.

One of the ironies in studying the health of physicians is that perfectionistic behaviors may be desired by patients and rewarded within the field while being personally expensive. Society's meat is the physician's poison (Gabbard 1985). On the positive side, perfectionism leads to thorough and comprehensive diagnostic efforts, the systemic ordering of laboratory tests to rule out the most exotic disorders, and detailed treatment planning that takes advantage of the latest innovations in treatment.

In some respects, the culture of medicine reflects the culture at large. North American society in many ways sanctions perfectionism. When an Olympic athlete is engaged in floor exercise or diving competition, the goal is a perfect 10.

Those who fall short of that perfect 10 are often relegated to journalistic phrases such as "This fine athlete unfortunately (or tragically) had to settle for only a bronze medal." Hence being the third best in the world is virtually equivalent to a failure.

Newsweek recently featured an article on pilot projects designed to reduce medical error rates to zero (Berwick and Leape 2006). The headline proclaimed, "Perfect is Possible." The story itself details the saga of a 2000 Robert Wood Johnson Foundation project that encouraged hospitals to "pursue perfection" in areas of reliability and safety. Physician and lay readers alike are thus encouraged to view perfection as a realistic goal. Hence the intrapsychic perfectionism of physicians is powerfully reinforced by the culture of medicine.

Despite these cultural sanctions, perfectionism is not actually adaptive. This personality trait has now been the subject of a growing body of research. It is a vulnerability factor for depression, burnout, suicide, and anxiety (Beevers and Miller 2004; Flett and Hewitt 2002; Hamilton and Schweitzer 2000). In fact, one study (Beevers and Miller 2004) demonstrated the impact of perfectionism to be both independent of and equal in significance to hopelessness, a factor commonly regarded as the best prospective predictor of suicidal ideation. Perfectionistic individuals often fail to differentiate the wish to excel from the desire to be perfect.

Many perfectionists believe that others will value them only if they are perfect. This particular belief is associated with both depression and suicide. Inherent in perfectionism is an element of pressure associated with a sense of both helplessness and hopelessness that can be translated into cognitive distortions such as, "The better I do, the better I'm expected to do" (Flett and Hewitt 2002).

The origins of perfectionism are not well understood. There appear to be multiple pathways (Flett and Hewitt 2002):

- Child factors—temperament, attachment style
- Parent factors—style of parenting, personality
- Environmental pressures—peers, culture, teachers

Clinical work with physicians who are perfectionistic often reveals a childhood conviction that they were not sufficiently valued or loved by their parents (Gabbard and Menninger 1988). They feel that if a transcendent state of flawlessness could ultimately be reached, the approval that they missed in childhood might finally be forthcoming. Hence low self-esteem is managed by pursuing perfection. This goal of perfection is complicated because satisfaction with real achievements is limited. Such individuals often feel a sense of fraudulence when they are recognized with an honor or award, as though they have deceived those who applaud their performance. Moreover, they are often tormented by an expectation that more will be demanded, and often they are correct in their assessment. More *is* demanded of them by colleagues and superiors, who view them as physicians who can be counted on to "get the job done, no matter what it takes."

The "driven" quality often seen in perfectionistic physicians is not linked to a genuine wish for pleasure. Rather, it is designed to gain relief from a tormenting conscience. Voltaire is said to have noted, "The perfect is the enemy of the good." Indeed, perfectionistic strivings rob the perfectionist of any gratification in more modest but laudable achievements.

Case Example

Dr. Simmons, a 29-year-old internal medicine resident, was in the process of applying for an endocrinology fellowship. She had come to psychotherapy because of a vague dissatisfaction with her life, both in work achievements and in relationships. She came to one therapy session with a letter of recommendation written by the chair of the internal medicine department. With a glum expression on her face, she handed the letter to her therapist and asked him to read it. As he read over the superlative letter, which praised the young resident in no uncertain terms, he was puzzled why she had such a dour expression. He asked her why she seemed so disappointed with such a glowing letter. Her response was succinct: "If he doesn't say I'm the best resident he's ever had in the program, I feel like a failure."

Excelling was not good enough for this physician. Only being the best—the most perfect resident in the program—would allow her to feel that she had succeeded. What the therapist knew, however, is that even if her chairman had said those words, she still would have been tormented by self-doubt. She would have said to herself that he really did not know her well enough, and she had simply deceived him.

Perfectionism is often accompanied by other compulsive traits (see Table 1–1). It rarely is a free-standing personality component. Perfectionistic physicians may also struggle with rigidity, stubbornness, and an inability to delegate tasks or to work with others unless they submit exactly to the physician's way of doing things. In addition, they may be excessively devoted to work and productivity to the exclusion of any leisure activities or friendships. Some end up being lonely and isolated people with no life outside of medicine.

A compulsive triad of self-doubt, guilt feelings, and an exaggerated sense of responsibility may be particularly typical of perfectionistic physicians (Gabbard 1985). The components of this triad account for a great deal of the suffering that physicians endure in the course of their practice. We consider each element of the triad separately for sake of elaboration, but they almost always occur in concert with one another.

To be sure, self-doubt, like perfectionism, has beneficial effects in that it leads physicians to be thorough in their diagnostic and treatment efforts. Pa-

TABLE 1–1. Compulsive traits common in physicians

Compulsive triad
    Self-doubt
    Guilt feelings
    Exaggerated sense of responsibility
Rigidity
Stubbornness
Inability to delegate
Excessive devotion to work, leading to neglect of relationships and leisure time
  activities
Perfectionism

tients want to have a compulsive and perfectionistic physician, because it provides peace of mind to the patient knowing that the physician is doing all that can be done to make an accurate diagnosis and prescribe optimal treatment. However, self-doubt is a double-edged sword because it can lead to chronic anxiety and torment for the physician who feels that living with uncertainty and lack of control is tantamount to failure.

Case Example

A 41-year-old radiology resident, Dr. Miller, was sent for a psychiatric evaluation because he was showing signs of burnout and depression. He explained to the psychiatrist conducting the evaluation that he had been a surgeon for 7 years prior to his radiology residency. He described a relentless pattern of self-doubt that had led him to switch specialties. After a complicated surgical procedure, he would find himself lying in bed at 3 A.M. staring at the ceiling and questioning his performance in the operating room. He would worry about whether he had closed the wound properly, whether he had left a 4 × 4 pad inside the patient, and whether he had maintained a sterile field. He also worried that a mistake would lead to a devastating malpractice suit that would destroy his reputation. He had hoped that switching to radiology would relieve him of this burden of self-doubt that accompanied patient care. However, now in his third year of residency, Dr. Miller realized that he was dealing with an intrapsychic state that was independent of his specialty. He was taking an inordinately long time to read magnetic resonance imaging (MRI) scans because he was preoccupied with what he termed "the million-dollar mistake." He elaborated that he and his fellow residents often discussed the consequences of misreading an MRI—namely, a lawsuit that would cost millions. As he explored the origins of this self-doubt in the evaluation, he noted that he grew up with perfectionistic parents who conveyed to him again and again that he was always falling short of their expectations.

Guilt feelings are also highly prevalent among physicians. The secret omnipotence of physicians may lead them to think that they are personally responsible for everything that happens to the patient, overlooking the fact that the practice of medicine always involves collaboration. Physicians can only make recommendations; patients must do their part by cooperating and following them. Moreover, almost all treatments have unforeseen consequences that cannot be predicted in advance. Many physicians deal with death anxiety and existential dread by attempting to outwit the Grim Reaper and triumph over death (Gabbard and Menninger 1988). The wish to control the course of disease and the trajectory of the patient's response to treatment frequently comes into direct conflict with the certainty of death and the doctor's impotence in the face of terminal illnesses. The physician may nevertheless have feelings of guilt and self-reproach about possible mistakes or misjudgments in the course of treatment when the patient dies.

Case Example

Dr. Green, a 34-year-old psychiatrist, was referred a 20-year-old patient who had made multiple suicide attempts related to diagnoses of depression and borderline personality disorder. The patient repeatedly told her psychiatrist that she was not really interested in treatment but was there only because her parents insisted that she get treatment. She insisted that she was utterly hopeless about her life ever improving, and she rarely talked about matters of real concern in her sessions with the psychiatrist. She had been through a whole series of antidepressants with very little response. She had even undergone electroconvulsive therapy, which also was ineffective in helping her with her suicidal ideation and depression. Because the suicidality was chronic, the psychiatrist never knew for sure when hospitalization should be considered. He recognized that if he hospitalized the patient, she would simply wait out the brief hospital stay and make the statements necessary to receive a discharge order from the inpatient attending. He also knew that the patient had had multiple hospitalizations and was unlikely to benefit from another. He explained to the patient that to continue the treatment as an outpatient, she would need to agree to call him before acting on her suicidal impulses. She reluctantly said she would.

After breaking up with a boyfriend, the patient was tearful during one particular session, and Dr. Green became more worried than usual about her. He asked her if she were feeling suicidal, and her response was, "Not any more than usual." He asked her if she could call him before acting on any impulses. She said she would. That night the patient's parents called the psychiatrist and informed him that she had hanged herself in their basement. Dr. Green responded with intense guilt feelings. For weeks he obsessed about what he should have done differently. Should he have insisted upon hospitalization? If she refused, should he have involuntarily committed her? Had he really given all the antidepressant medications a full trial at sufficiently high dosages? Should he have worked more closely with the family? Did he miss signs that the patient's chronic suicidality had dipped into acute suicidality? He even seriously considered leaving the profession because of his lack of control in such situations and his feelings that he might not be competent enough to treat severely disturbed patients.

Despite colleagues' reassurance that he had conducted a competent and even heroic treatment, his guilt feelings did not subside for many months. He could not accept the notion that some psychiatric illnesses are terminal and will not respond to any kind of treatment. Colleagues who knew him empathized and tried to explain that certain patients who are determined to kill themselves will not collaborate in any treatment effort.

An exaggerated sense of responsibility is clearly related to both self-doubt and guilt feelings. Professionalism demands a sense of responsibility and ethical conduct, of course, and physicians must be dedicated to their patients. Moreover, as in the case with this young psychiatrist, physicians are not entirely responsible for the outcomes of their patients. Most of medicine is palliative, except for certain infectious diseases and surgical procedures (Gabbard and Menninger 1988). Some outcomes are not preventable. Psychiatrists in particular may have difficulty accepting the idea that *some* psychiatric disorders in *some* patients are terminal. Moreover, research suggests that psychiatrists may have more death anxiety than other specialists (Viswanathan 1996) and therefore may do poorly when patients kill themselves. Also, the culture of malpractice litigation reinforces the idea that someone must be responsible for a bad outcome and that that person must pay for it. Given the heroics performed in some medical centers around end-of-life care, at least some trainees feel dreadful if a patient dies under their watch. An expected and perhaps inevitable outcome is seen as a "bad outcome."

Physicians in training strive to practice error-free medicine, so any mistake takes its toll. Frequency of self-perceived medical errors was recorded prospectively in a cohort study of internal medicine residents at the Mayo Clinic (West et al. 2006). Thirty-four percent of participants made at least one major medical error during the study period. Self-perceived mistakes were associated with a statistically significant decrease in quality of life and worsened measures in all domains of burnout. They were also associated with screening positive for depression. In addition, increased burnout in all domains and reduced empathy were associated with increased odds of self-perceived error in the *following* 3 months. The researchers concluded that personal distress and decreased empathy are associated with increased odds of future self-perceived errors, suggesting that perceived errors and distress may be related to one another in a vicious circle.

Most of what is known about the psychological characteristics of physicians comes from clinical anecdotes based on treating or evaluating physicians. However, a small body of research contributes to our knowledge. Vaillant et al. (1972) followed a cohort of young men from college age throughout the life cycle. They noted that self-doubt was a characteristic that distinguished physicians from control subjects. The intensive training, the string of credentials, the diplomas on their walls, and the authority imbued upon them by society often are elements of a defensive posture designed to ward off the daily reminders of fallibility (Gabbard and Menninger 1988). However, no amount of achievement or success eradicates the underlying self-doubt.

Vaillant's group also noted that physicians with primary responsibility for patient care were more likely to have emotionally impoverished childhoods compared with nonphysicians in the cohort. The investigators suggested that frontline practitioners may be giving care and attention to their patients as a way of giving to others what they did not receive when they themselves were children. This study also indicated that physicians may defend against anger and longings for dependency through reaction formation—in other words, they give to others as a way of denying their own neediness and anger. Selfless efforts to care for others reassure them that their own dependency and smoldering resentment are under control. Many physicians are prone to attribute any difficulties they have to the stress of practice, however, the study conducted by Vaillant and colleagues suggests that the reverse is true. Work stress usually becomes a significant factor because of an underlying vulnerability in physicians. A study of 142 Scottish medical students (both male and female) during their first undergraduate year and their senior residency year (Baldwin et al. 1997) reached similar conclusions. They found that the feeling of being overwhelmed was not significantly correlated with long hours worked.

A classic and time-honored study of 800 gifted men (Terman 1954) showed that physicians as a group tend to feel inferior. Insecurity seems pervasive, and physicians may seek approval through more work, more achievement, and more triumph over disease. Of course, this study is more than a half-century old and involved male physicians exclusively. We must be cautious about extrapolating from these findings to the psychology of contemporary physicians. Nevertheless, the lack of self-confidence rings true across the decades. The narcissism often attributed to physicians may be warranted, but it is wise to remember that the efforts to puff oneself up and impress others may be a defense against feelings of insecurity and self-doubt.

The Culture of Medicine

These psychological characteristics, certainly found in most physicians, lead to a specific approach to work. Dedication to the patient is accompanied by conscientiousness about accurate diagnosis and the best treatment available. The exaggerated sense of responsibility may lead to long work hours and difficulty delegating coverage to other physicians. Similarly, there may be a severe restriction of leisure time as a result of this devotion to work. In one sample of 100 physicians (Krakowski 1982), only 16 reported watching television for pleasure or attending theatre or concerts. Only 10 physicians in the sample regularly took off time to relax, and only 11 took vacations exclusively for vacation's sake. Even though this study is more than a quarter-century old, its findings are still relevant today. Indeed, time devoted to oneself and pleasurable pursuits may be regarded as selfish and neglectful of one's duty to patients and the profession.

These workaholic patterns appear to be well established by the time that young physicians are residents. In 2003 the Accreditation Council for Graduate Medical Education mandated work hour limits because of evidence that exhaustion compromised performance. The new standards permitted 30 consecutive hours of work and 80 hours per week. However, a national cohort study of 4,015 interns in U.S. residency programs (Landrigan et al. 2006) indicated that the hour limits were regularly violated in the first year after implementation. Eighty-three percent of study interns reported working hours that were noncompliant for at least 1 month in the year after the limits were introduced. The investigators noted that there was a widespread perception among physicians that fatigue is not a problem—in spite of the evidence. They also noted that the culture of medicine is often antagonistic to work hour limits, and senior physicians have been outspoken in expressing clear disapproval of them. Many agree that patient care is compromised when responsibility repeatedly shifts from one resident to another (Okie 2007). Patients may be unclear about who is in charge of their treatment.

As suggested by these findings, the preexisting character traits of those who become doctors are further enhanced by the culture of medicine in academic training centers. A well-known surgeon at a leading medical school spoke to the first-year students as they began their training. He advised them that they should plan on giving up all leisure time pursuits as they embarked on their medical careers because from that time on, all their pleasures would come from the practice of medicine. A stark message of this nature delivered by a figure endowed with awe and respect has extraordinary influence. It inaugurates an acculturation experience in which students observe role models who are devoted to the practice of medicine to the extent that all other interests fade into the background. They see professors who arrive at the hospital at 5 A.M. for rounds and do not go home until 10 P.M.

When the students reach their clinical clerkships, the house officers, who are only a few years older than the students, also have a powerful impact. Despite exhausting schedules, an up-to-date knowledge of the literature is essential. Residents may expect the students to have read the latest issue of *The New England Journal of Medicine* and apply the knowledge from a clinical trial reported in that issue to the treatment of a patient who has just been admitted to the hospital. A strong ethic of responsibility is inculcated as well. Skepticism is conveyed about turning over the management of a patient to someone else who is covering for the primary physician. To win the approval of the attending physicians and house officers, students learn they must run the extra mile and strive toward perfection. Training often underemphasizes the patient's responsibility in maintaining health, lending credence to the notion that the physicians must bear the total responsibility. The healthcare industry at large, however, is now exploring the role played by the patient's personal responsibility for health (Steinbrook 2006).

The culture of medicine also provides an irreducible experience of shame and humiliation. Much of the acculturation experience occurs with an "audience" of peers, interns, residents, and attending faculty. When a student is asked to identify the three components of Hasselbach's Triangle in the operating room, a host of observers are watching and listening as the student attempts to prove his or her knowledge of surgical anatomy. On medical rounds, a sea of white coats goes from one room to the next, and the attending physician may unexpectedly ask a student to recite the clinical manifestations of Cushing's syndrome. A failure to respond in these settings with the correct answers often leads to a devastating experience of humiliating exposure. Whether or not the attending physician berates the student for not knowing the answer, students in these situations are often highly self-critical and feel ashamed of being less than perfect in their medical knowledge. They feel like losers or failures, and the result is to throw themselves headlong into even more compulsive memorization of what they need to know to be a competent physician.

When the newly minted specialist leaves residency or fellowship and enters the world of medical practice, the culture of medicine continues to shape the values, behavior, and thinking of the young physician. The extraordinary premiums paid for malpractice insurance in certain specialties, and the widely publicized consequences of malpractice suits, hang over the physician's head like a cloud. This ever-present threat leads the physician to be more perfectionistic, more compulsive, and more diligent in his or her efforts to practice a brand of medicine that is beyond reproach. Primary relationships and the raising of children may be relegated to one's spouse or to an au pair. Many physicians enter into a psychology of postponement (Gabbard and Menninger 1989) at this point in their careers. They feel that they must place their practice first to establish themselves. They may need to spend time in the doctors' lounge at the hospital on Saturday and Sunday morning to get to know other physicians and to cultivate referral sources. They may feel that they must respond to requests for consultation as quickly as possible so they are seen as conscientious and prompt. They worry that failure to respond rapidly may lead the referral source to look elsewhere for a consultant.

When they talk to their partner or spouse during this period of time—in a way that is intended to be reassuring—the conversation often sounds something like this:

> I'm sorry that I'm not more available to you now, but this is only a temporary situation. Once I'm established in the community, I will be home a great deal more. I will spend more time with you (and the children) at that point. Right now, though, I have to make sure that all my colleagues know I am committed to medicine and will be available to them when they need me.

Many spouses and partners have heard similar promises during medical school, residency, and fellowships. They begin to grow cynical and may even give up on their fantasies that things will one day be different. Ultimately the psychology of postponement may be revealed as a psychology of avoidance (Gabbard and Menninger 1989). Varying degrees of estrangement and isolation result from this pattern of behavior as a result of the physician's greater comfort with work than with the spontaneous intimacy of primary relationships at home.

The Female Physician

In North America today, medical students are roughly equally divided by gender. Female students must have many of the same psychological features as their male counterparts to gain entrance into the highly competitive medical schools to which they apply. Nevertheless, research indicates that there are gender differences in the way that identities develop. Gilligan (1982) noted that boys develop autonomy by separating themselves from their mothers, whereas separation and autonomy are not nearly as important for girls. They develop their female identities in close association with their mothers. Boys tend to seek greater independence and self-sufficiency, whereas girls value relatedness, affiliation, and emotional closeness. These findings are not necessarily applicable to every individual, of course, but they represent large group differences that may be significant in the way that female physicians practice medicine and also in the way that their greater numbers may affect the culture of medicine.

Some of these gender differences are reflected in recent research about the differences between male and female physicians. For example, a study of the malpractice experience of 9,250 physicians (Taragin et al. 1992) found that male physicians were three times as likely to be in the high claims group as female physicians, even after adjustment for other demographic variables. The investigators suggested that the most likely explanation was that women interact more effectively with their patients and foster relationships that are preventative against lawsuits.

In a landmark study from the Society of General Internal Medicine (SGIM) Career Satisfaction Study Group, McMurray et al. (2000) found a number of significant differences in the practices of male and female physicians. Female physicians were significantly more likely to report satisfaction with their specialty and with patient and colleague relationships compared with their male counterparts. However, they were less likely to be satisfied with autonomy, relationships with the community, pay, and resources. Female physicians also saw more female patients and more patients with complex psychosocial problems. The female doctors reported needing 36% more time than allotted to provide quality care for new patients or consultations, compared with only 21% more time needed by men. As noted in other studies, the mean income for women was approximately $22,000 less than that of men. Women also had 1.6 times the odds of reporting burnout compared with men. In fact, lack of workplace control predicted burnout in women but not in men.

In a subsequent study presented at the 2005 Association of American Medical Colleges Conference, Horner-Ibler (noted in Croasdale 2005) reported results that were intended to build on the SGIM Study Group report. Surveying 420 primary care physicians in Illinois, New York, and Wisconsin, as well as 2,500 of their patients, they found that women physicians were twice as likely to report high levels of stress and feelings of burnout compared with male counterparts. They also expressed a wish to have more time for patients and felt more at odds with the values of the organizations in which they worked than men. They tended to see patients with highly complex cases that required more time, and they wanted more family-friendly workplaces.

Similar findings emerged from a study of 2,398 Canadian physicians regarding their practices and attitudes toward healthcare issues (Williams et al. 1990). Women tended to organize and manage their practices differently. For example, women preferred group over solo practice and also gravitated toward community health centers and health service organizations. Men were more inclined to be in solo practices and underrepresented in community health centers and health service organizations. As in American studies, the incomes of women physicians were significantly lower than those of men. The investigators noted that women physicians often have a double workload as both professionals and family caregivers, so that their stresses may be experienced differently than those of men. In another Canadian survey (Woodward et al. 1996), for example, half of the respondents had children at home. Women physicians with children at home spent significantly fewer hours on professional activities than did men. When the male physicians were compared with other male physicians who did not have children, their hours of professional activity were similar. In addition to the extra burden that women physicians carry for the rearing of children, they also are often responsible for aging parents and parents-in-law. They are frequently viewed as nurturers who will take care of the needs of other family members while men continue to spend the majority of their time in the workplace. Hence female physicians often end up feeling that they are spending their days giving to others without any replenishment for themselves.

One disconcerting sign of increased vulnerability in female physicians is their suicide rate. Whereas the male suicide rate is more than four times that of females in the general population, the suicide rate of female physicians is as high as the rate of male physicians (Silverman 2000). No one knows the reasons for this alarming finding. In part, it may be related to the higher prevalence of depression in women. However, many speculate that it may be related, in part, to the extra domestic burdens typically shouldered by women physicians.

Female physicians may also undergo greater levels of harassment during the course of training than their male counterparts. In addition, when women physicians become pregnant, they may become the objects of resentment to their colleagues in the training program. They may feel guilty about causing an increase in the number of on-call nights for colleagues because they are taking time off for parental leave.

Despite the challenges faced by women physicians, evidence is growing that they have contributed to a veritable backlash against the traditional macho ethos of medical training and practice. Women are less likely to buy into the notion that work comes before everything else. They naturally seek more balance to their lives because of the need to have time to care for children at home. In a comprehensive study of female physicians in the United States, Frank et al. (1998) found that women doctors have generally good health habits when compared with other women from comparable socioeconomic groups. They smoke less, drink moderately, and attend to health screening procedures. To some extent, female medical students and house officers have served as role models for their male colleagues, who see them setting limits on the demands of their work and devoting themselves equally to family and personal lives. We are now seeing evidence that both male and female physicians are in the midst of a generational shift in attitude toward work.

In a study of the specialty choices of U.S. medical students graduating between 1996 and 2003, Dorsey et al. (2005) found that both women and men are more inclined to choose a specialty with controllable hours than in the past. Clearly, men are starting to look for more of a work/life balance. These investigators found that the percentage of women seeking specialties with controllable lifestyles, such as ophthalmology, psychiatry, and radiology, increased by 18 percentage points. Their male counterparts also increased their interest in those specialties by 17 percentage points.

A similar study looking at the specialty choice of medical students between 1990 and 2003 (Lambert and Holmboe 2005) found that physicians of both sexes had a declining interest in specialties in which there was not a work/family life balance, such as family medicine. In 1995 18.9% of women and 15.2% of men chose family medicine residencies; 8 years later, these percentages had declined to 10% and 6.1%, respectively. This shift in priorities related to guarding the balance of work and family life has changed not only the selection of specialties to some degree but also the choice of practice setting. Physicians today are more likely to ask about coverage arrangements in group practice, weekend duty, night call, and regular hours than in years past. Moreover, groups attempting to recruit first-rate physicians who are completing their residencies or fellowships know that they must take such considerations into account to attract the physicians they seek to add to their practices.

Despite these changes that are on the horizon, many physicians still struggle with guilt feelings regarding efforts to lead a balanced life. One 35-year-old psychiatrist who went back to part-time practice after maternity leave put it this way: "If I stay at home with my baby, I feel guilty about leaving my patients unattended. But when I am with my patients, I feel like a bad mother who is neglecting her child. It's a no-win situation." Often the perfectionism of physicians applies as much to parenthood as it does to work. Physician parents may want to provide the ideal setting for their children and realize it is impossible as long as they continue to practice. Women physicians may experience more guilt feelings because of an upbringing in which a woman's main role was in the home. Hence there are often conflicting identifications at work that create intrapsychic conflict in women physicians. In any case, the psychology of the female physician has much in common with that of the male physician, but a greater vulnerability to burnout, depression, and suicide must be taken into account.

Key Points

- Influences inherent in the culture of medicine interact with preexisting psychological characteristics of those who enter medicine to pose a set of occupational hazards for most physicians.
- Perfectionism and other compulsive personality traits are present in the majority of physicians and contribute to a vulnerability to depression, suicide, anxiety, and burnout.
- A compulsiveness triad of self-doubt, guilt feelings, and an exaggerated sense of responsibility is particularly problematic for many physicians.
- The culture of medicine in academic medical centers and the threat of malpractice suits exacerbate preexisting psychological tendencies toward perfectionism and compulsiveness and contribute to experiences of shame and humiliation during training.
- The psychology of postponement may relate to difficulties in intimate relationships among physicians, who may prefer work to emotional closeness.
- Although female physicians have similar psychological features to male physicians, they tend to value relatedness, affiliation, and intimacy more than do men.
- Female physicians are less likely to be sued but are more prone to burnout than male physicians and have equivalent rates of suicide.
- Recent data on specialty choices of medical students indicate that a generational shift is occurring, among both male and female physicians, in terms of prioritizing the balance of work and family.

Minority Physicians (Racial, Ethnic, Sexual Orientation) and International Medical Graduates

In Chapter 1 we emphasized that psychological characteristics of physicians interact with the culture of medicine. However, the psychology of the physician is also influenced by culture in the broader sense—the customs, outlook, and way of life of particular groups within North American society. Despite the visible pluralism of North American physicians, there has been a tendency in the field of physician health to study and treat physicians as though they were a unitary entity (with the exception of gender). Like the population that doctors serve, physicians are a mosaic of race, ethnicity, and culture.

In this chapter, we discuss what is unique about physicians who are members of minority groups and/or who are International Medical Graduates (IMGs). A detailed literature search yielded few empirical studies of these physicians and their mental health. Although women in medicine are no longer deemed a minority, the Women Physicians' Health Study stands alone as the largest and most scientifically sound status report on U.S. female doctors (Frank et al. 1998). As noted in Chapter 1 ("The Psychology of Physicians and the Culture of Medicine"), results showed that women physicians report generally good health habits, and although the demographics included white, African American, Asian American, and Hispanic physicians, there were no specific illness vulnerabilities in minority physicians.

African American Physicians

There is a dearth of published literature on the health of black physicians. One paper, albeit old, reported a link between obesity and hypertension in black physicians (Neser et al. 1986). No studies of African American physicians were presented at the past two International Conferences on Physician Health in 2004 and 2006. In the medical student literature, minority students report more stress than their nonminority colleagues (Anderson 1991) and a greater sense of their lives being out of their control after 1 year of medical school (Pyskoty et al. 1990). Black students appear to use drugs less frequently than majority medical students (Forney et al. 1988). One study of impairment in black physicians found that they were more likely to abuse tranquilizers than any other drug (Carter 1989). We have no empirical data on the prevalence of mood disorders in African American physicians.

Webb (2000) described special challenges for African American medical students. Racism is common in medicine. Black students report mistreatment to a greater degree than do majority students (Richardson et al. 1997). If the black student is not attending a historically black medical school, identity development can be thwarted by having few African American physician role models and lack of support from the majority culture. Furthermore, black students struggle with pursuing the Afrocentric view (meeting the needs of the group) because it conflicts with the Eurocentric view (achievement in individual pursuits) (Post and Weddington 1997). Pressure to give back to their community and the underserved may overload the student. African American students describe feeling "different" (and frustrated) when it comes to having fun, dating (especially for female students), coping with financial strain, finding a church, and shopping for certain foods and hair products or stylists.

It is always salutary not only to delineate problems but also to highlight strengths. Results of structured telephone interviews with 50 black physicians across the country (Webb et al. 2000) identified "secrets of success" that reflect features of the African-American culture.

- Know your legacy: pay attention to the wisdom of elders, especially other African American physicians
- Draw strength from the community
- Draw on spiritual strength
- Be in control of your response to racism
- Maintain who you are and where you are going
- Adapt quickly
- Get organized and "just do it"

Case Example

Dr. Thomas was a 33-year-old black physician who was a junior resident in cardiology when he came to see a psychiatrist. He was quite depressed. Given the history of a previous illness in medical school and a significant family history of mood disorders (and suicide), he was diagnosed as having major depressive disorder, recurrent type. He was restarted on the same antidepressant that had been helpful for his earlier depression. Within 10 days, he was beginning to feel better. With improvement of his mood and cognition, his psychiatrist was able to obtain valuable historical information and the psychosocial factors at work in the precipitation of his clinical symptoms.

First, Dr. Thomas felt very isolated in his department. He was the only black resident, and there were no faculty members—academic or clinical—who were black. "In fact, I'm it. There are minority nurses, aides, laboratory technicians, clerical staff, and housekeeping personnel—but not one is black. I've had a couple of black patients and that's been refreshing. I think I'm a bit of an oddity in this city." Having attended a mostly minority student medical school, Dr. Thomas experienced the work setting as very foreign. Second, he was single and good-looking. "I get a lot of attention from the nurses and others at work. I've done a lot of dating. It's great for the ego. Most of the women ask me out. Easy sex too. But there's no intimacy. It's very empty. And very lonely." Third, Dr. Thomas felt dismissed for what he called his humanistic side. "I've always been interested in storytelling. It's part of my black heritage, going back so many generations. This is what attracted me to medicine. I would have pursued psychiatry, but I'm in cardiology because heart disease is rampant in my family, and I want to contribute to research into this killer. But my attendings are not interested in the nuts and bolts of my patients' lives. They've been very critical of the time I spend at the bedside and my presentations at rounds [he became teary at this point]…that hurts."

Dr. Thomas found psychotherapy helpful. He explored at length his ambivalence about being a racial minority health professional in his field. On the one hand, he enjoyed the attention and distinction. On the other, he hated the isolation and loneliness. He discussed notions of belonging and authentic representation as a member of a nondominant group (Griffith 2005). As a solo black man, he wanted to represent his group well, but this effort also felt like a burden. His aloneness as a black physician and the criticism that he received for his clinical style with patients were very painful for him. He felt that he did not belong, and he chastised himself for obsessively worrying about this, given that academically he was so highly regarded. He felt stereotyped as a black sex object by the women whom he dated and who flirted with him. This too eroded his self-esteem. Although it took awhile for him to trust his white psychiatrist, he felt validated for his musings and found that his therapist could empathize with his anguish. Like so many troubled physicians, he wondered if he was being self-indulgent. Most important, his psychiatrist's interest in detailed history-taking and in knowing patients in depth resonated with how he practiced cardiology and his own personal interest in his patients' lives. Reflecting on the treatment, Dr. Thomas said, "The antidepressant got me functioning again, but my healing is a result of these sessions."

Primm (2006), writing about African American patients, highlighted important cultural issues in assessment and treatment. Her notions of racial consciousness, self-identity, self-determination, family patterns, black versus African American self-designation, assimilation, nonverbal communication and language, eye contact, gestures and the cross-racial therapeutic relationship, and much more have great relevance and meaning for mental health professionals who treat African American physicians.

Hispanic Physicians

The health of Hispanic physicians has not been extensively studied, with the exception of work-related stress and professional satisfaction. In a national sample of physicians, 134 of the 2,217 respondents were Hispanics (Glymour et al. 2004). Among the findings, it was reconfirmed that minority physicians treat a more demanding and underserved patient base than white physicians. Hispanic physicians reported significantly higher job and career satisfaction compared with white physicians but no significant difference in stress.

Despite the heterogeneity of Hispanic minorities in the United States, there are similarities in the organizations of their local worlds (Canive et al. 2001). Extrapolating from the general population to the Hispanic physician population may be risky but yet illustrative in understanding how we might better treat this group of doctors. What follows are some important principles that have been outlined by Canive et al. (2001):

- *Language proficiency.* If the physician-patient is not completely fluent in English, switching from Spanish to English, speaking in a disjointed or excited manner, or gesturing a lot, one must appreciate what is culturally normative and not erroneously read psychopathology into the assessment. Emotionally laden communications are often better expressed in the mother tongue.
- *The centrality of family.* Members of a family are expected to support one another, emotionally and materially, and usually unconditionally. An "overinvolved" mother of a 40-year-old single Hispanic physician son living at home may not see how she could be thwarting his need for separation-individuation.
- *Religion and spirituality.* Many Hispanic physicians are practicing Catholics. Depending on their ancestry and/or country of origin, they may also incorporate folk and American Indian or African rituals into their beliefs. Therapists who treat Hispanic physicians must not only respect these values but also determine how they may be used in a protective and/or restorative way in the treatment plan.
- *"Machismo" history. Machismo* is a noun of Spanish origin and refers to prominently exhibited or excessive masculinity. Hispanic male physicians will vary enormously in how easily they accept professional help, especially psychiatric help, and from whom. They may be ashamed of being ill and will

deny or rationalize the degree of their pain or dysfunction. Their marriages will vary from classically traditional to dual career. They may not be able to talk about sexual difficulties. They may feel deeply humiliated if they fail their board examinations or are struggling financially compared with their medical peers.

- *Somatization.* It is not pejorative to suggest that some Hispanic physicians may manifest stress and emotional distress with a range of bodily symptoms (Gonzalez et al. 2001). This is a culturally bound idiomatic way of communicating. Because of the importance of the supernatural in Hispanic culture, it is not inappropriate or insulting to ask even the most scientifically oriented physicians about their views on such matters.
- *Treatment models.* Depending on the physician, individual and insight-oriented therapy, directive counseling, and cognitive-behavioral approaches may all be helpful. Psychoeducation, especially with the family, can be useful as well. Intensely loving and concerned family members might be more responsive to backing away a little if they are seen as simply caring and devoted, not enmeshed or undermining.

Although these principles can be unifying, therapists must always remember that the cultural context of a symptomatic physician from Spain may be very different than that of a physician from Chile or El Salvador. Each brings a unique story to the treatment setting.

Asian American Physicians

Asian Americans are the third largest minority group in the United States, comprising different ethnic subgroups with diverse languages and dialects, religious beliefs, immigration patterns, socioeconomic statuses, and patterns of seeking healthcare (Du 2006). Within the Asian American population, the most common groups are Chinese, Filipino, Asian Indian, Vietnamese, Korean, and Japanese. Asian American physicians are represented by all of these, with most being Chinese, Filipino, and Asian Indian. There are no data on the prevalence of mental illness, including substance abuse and dependence, in Asian American doctors.

When the clinician is assessing an Asian American physician, it is prudent to employ principles outlined in DSM-IV-TR's "Outline for Cultural Formulation" (American Psychiatric Association 2000a). It aids the clinician in at least four ways to obtain a rich biopsychosocial impression and to implement treatment (Group for the Advancement of Psychiatry, Committee on Cultural Psychiatry 2002):

1. Evaluation of the patient's cultural/ethnic identity
2. Cultural explanations of the illness
3. Cultural factors related to the psychosocial environment and levels of functioning
4. Cultural elements of the doctor–patient relationship

Arising from and incorporating much of the published literature on this matter (Du 2006), the following principles and suggestions are salient when assessing and treating Asian American physicians:

- Attempt to understand the current state of the physician's cultural identity. What is their sense of belonging and identification with other members of the group? How traditional? How assimilated?
- Listen to self-references. A more traditional Asian American doctor may prefer to be referred to as Chinese American or Indo-American. A physician whose family has been here for one or more generations prefers to be called American.
- Ask about religion and religious philosophies. The faiths of Asian Americans include Confucianism, Taoism, Buddhism, Roman Catholicism, Protestantism, Hinduism, Islam, and more.
- Appreciate hierarchy in the family with respect for elders and firstborn males. Watch for face-saving as a protective mechanism. Understand that open disagreement with treating physicians is unusual.
- When assessing the patient's personality, consider the following: Even the most extroverted, outwardly confident and assertive physician may ascribe to traditional Asian virtues of modesty, decorum, humility, and being polite. The needs of one's immediate and extended family (or community) supersede self-interest.
- Maintain a broad perspective. Asian American physicians often respect (if not embrace) non-Western theories of illness and treatments. This includes various spiritual and holistic measures, herbal medicines, acupuncture, Tai Chi, morita therapy, and more.
- Be aware of how psychotropic medications affect Asian Americans by studying ethnopsychopharmacology (Smith 2006).
- Remember that anxiety and depression may manifest somatically rather than be felt and expressed in psychological language.
- Respect the many determinants of identity. One's culture may eclipse the physician's training in American psychiatry as a medical student or resident.
- Remember that many medical students and physicians will live at home until they get married. Separation-individuation is different for Asian American physicians than for their classmates or colleagues. When they marry they may live with one or the other's parents, or they will unquestionably have elderly parents cohabiting within their home.

- Appreciate family dynamics. Younger physicians may be in conflict with their parents for wanting to live apart from them. Distress over this conflict may contribute to a mood disorder, an eating disorder, or acting-out behaviors. Because of assimilation and small numbers of members with their own ethnic identity group, many will inter-date or intermarry. This can be wrenching for all parties.
- Watch for and be empathic with homosexuality struggles. Gay or lesbian Asian American physicians have even more challenges than their non-Asian counterparts. A homosexual relationship is considered to be sexual lust in Buddhism, a breach of the harmony of yin and yang in Taoism, and a sin in Christianity (Nakajima et al. 1996). For some families, it is a source of shame to the family's name.
- Keep an open mind about attitudes toward mental illness and its treatments. Asian American physicians are on a continuum regarding embracing psychiatric care. The more traditional, the greater the delay, and the sicker they will be when they present. Stigma is as strong as in American physicians, but that said, many young Asian American physicians of today easily and quickly come for help. Attitudes toward medication and psychotherapy vary tremendously. It is important to fight stereotypic thinking that Asian American physicians prefer cognitive-behavioral approaches to psychodynamic ones.
- Understand the extent of embarrassment and guardedness at the beginning of treatment. Because domestic violence is not uncommon in many Asian cultures, one must ask about this when assessing physicians and their marriages. Shame and family secrets preclude open discussion until there is a therapeutic alliance. This sense of privacy and humiliation may cloak information about teenagers who are sexually acting out or abusing drugs, problem drinking in the doctor-patient, divorce, or gambling and other addictions.
- Examine countertransference when treating Asian American physicians. Recognize that cultural stereotyping in trying to understand your patient often occurs (Comas-Diaz and Jacobsen 1991). When the therapist and patient share the same ethnocultural background, there is a risk of intraethnic countertransference, which may include feelings of survivor guilt (treating physicians who are refugees or who have been victims of torture), overidentification, and defensive distancing (to ward off feelings of anxiety, grief, anger). Interethnic countertransference (when therapist and patient are of different ethnicities) includes inappropriate exploration of values and customs (that can be perceived as voyeuristic or intellectualized), guilt grounded in perceived collusion with the oppressive majority, cultural myopia and denial of significance, and aggression based on unrecognized prejudice.

Case Example

Dr. Tan and his wife consulted a psychiatrist for marital therapy. They are both Chinese. He is a radiologist, she is a realtor. They are the parents of a 2-year-old child. "My wife wants me to move out. I don't want to. I didn't know she was so upset until she said this last week," said Dr. Tan. Mrs. Tan replied, "My husband is a very mixed up man. He works hard all day and surfs the Internet all evening. He says he is relaxing. Does relaxing take 5 hours? Does relaxing mean visiting porn sites? Is it not more important to play with your son or give him a bath at night than to read Chinese news online or obsessively check the stock market or look at naked women?"

They both agreed that things had been good at home until the latter months of pregnancy. Mrs. Tan had gained a lot of weight, and there had been worry about diabetes and pre-eclampsia. Although not depressed postpartum, she was weak. Mrs. Tan said, "In Chinese tradition, the first month is very important for recovery. You must eat well and pay close attention to nutrition. You should rest and get good sleep too. My cousin stayed with us for that month to help me. But my husband, being Chinese, should know better than to bug me for sex during that first month. And because he is a doctor, shouldn't he know that I am sore in my sexual area? So now he tells me it is my fault that he visits porn sites. I am the cause, he says. This began during that first month."

This example pinpoints a reference to a cultural or ethnic norm uttered by one of the spouses in marital therapy. The therapist must take note and ask the spouse, in this case the husband, if that is his understanding of the Chinese tradition as well. If he concurs, then he will explain himself in that context. If he does not concur or pleads ignorance, his explanation may have a different meaning to his wife. It may still seem to her that it was very insensitive of her husband to want to be sexual in the first postpartum month, but maybe less so. Whether the therapist is of the same culture or different becomes relevant if there is perceived collusion with one or the other patient.

Gay, Lesbian, Bisexual, and Transgendered Physicians

Given the long history of homophobia in our society, including our medical schools, it is impossible to know how many physicians in the United States are lesbian, gay, bisexual, or transgendered (LGBT). What we do know is that there has been a sea change in the visibility and openness about sexual orientation and gender identity over the past generation of physicians. This reflects both a societal and a medical culture transformation that has come about through advancement of knowledge and education. In medicine, this process began in 1973, when the diagnosis of homosexuality was removed from the official diagnostic manual of the American Psychiatric Association. Yet even today psychiatrists continue their efforts to ensure that gay and lesbian people are not discriminated against when applying to psychoanalytic institutes and that so-called reparative therapy (or conversion therapy) is deemed antithetical to psychological growth, if not actually damaging.

Studies show that LGBT populations, in addition to having the same basic health needs as the general population, experience health disparities and barriers related to sexual orientation and/or gender identity or expression (Gay and Lesbian Medical Association 2006). Many avoid or delay care or receive inappropriate or inferior care because of perceived or real homophobia, biphobia, transphobia, and discrimination by healthcare professionals and institutions. In one study, lesbian physicians were about four times more likely than heterosexual women physicians to report harassment related to sexual orientation, primarily during training and medical practice (Brogan et al. 1999).

With regard to mood disorders, there is no empirical evidence that these illnesses are more common in LGBT physicians than in heterosexual physicians. Can being a gay physician be a psychosocial stressor that contributes to depression? Absolutely, especially in a branch of medicine that is still quite homophobic; when a gay physician is struggling with unresolved and internalized homophobia that generates anxiety, guilt, and self-hatred; or if bisexual physicians find themselves unaccepted by their straight and gay colleagues. Regarding substance abuse and dependence, there are data showing that LGBT individuals are overrepresented in recovery programs, but this research is mixed. Whether this finding extends to LGBT physicians is uncertain, because physician health programs tend not to ask about or record sexual orientation, and many physicians would not disclose this anyway. We know that many physicians who drink too much, self-prescribe, and/or use street drugs are invisible. They have never sought treatment voluntarily nor been identified as impaired in their work. How many such individuals might be LGBT is not known.

What about suicide? Suicide research has identified gay and lesbian individuals, especially adolescents, at higher risk for suicide. This includes black male adolescents, a group already at risk. Given the shroud of secrecy and stigma that surrounds physician suicide, any estimation of rates characterized by sexual orientation would be speculative.

When we examine relationship strain and demise, there are no data for LGBT physician couples. Although there is research on divorce in physicians (Doherty and Burge 1989; Sotile and Sotile 2000), gay and lesbian doctors are not permitted to get married except in Massachusetts and Canada. The committed relationships of gay and lesbian individuals are more akin to their heterosexual married colleagues than different (Myers 1994). With regard to the sexual orientation of the children of LGBT parents, research has consistently shown that the offspring of gay male and lesbian couples are no more likely to become gay or lesbian themselves. These data can safely be extended to LGBT physician couples.

Self-disclosure of one's sexual orientation and its extension—going public—is usually connected with the notion of societal acceptance. However, despite the openness of many gay and lesbian physicians in North America, many have stories to tell about how unaccepted or judged they have felt by their medical colleagues. Some are selectively open. They may be out to their classmates but not to attending physicians. They are out to family and close friends but not workmates. They are open at work but not with their parents.

Much has been written about the travails of LGBT physicians in finding gay-friendly healthcare (Gay and Lesbian Medical Association 2006). With reference to educating mental health professionals about treating LGBT physicians with respect, especially thorough interviewing, the following suggestions are offered:

- Do not assume sexual orientation based on appearance, voice, mannerisms, marital status, or branch of medicine. Your patient will be very attuned to this and may not be honest with you or make an attempt to correct you.

  > Tim, a 30-year-old urology resident, never did disclose to his psychiatrist who treated him for depression for almost 3 years that he was gay. Or conversely, Sally who was a resident in orthopedic surgery, had to repeatedly remind her therapist that her partner was her husband. She said "I know I'm androgynous looking, but I just wish health professionals would not assume I'm gay and simply ask first."

- Do not ask about sexual orientation, unless it is crucial to do so. If your LGBT patient is comfortable and trusting of you, that information will be volunteered. This may happen in the first visit or after a therapeutic alliance is formed.
- Use gender-neutral language. Rather than asking if the physician is married, which may be experienced as insensitive or insulting, you can ask, "Are you in a committed relationship with anyone?"
- Be careful not to project your own comfort with homosexuality on to your LGBT physician-patients. They may have a lot of internalized homophobia. It is important that they be allowed to ventilate about this without the therapist quickly challenging their harsh thoughts or educating or normalizing. Remember that LGBT physicians are a mix of human beings with very different backgrounds, religious affiliations, and ethnic cultural beliefs that have shaped them. What is more important is that the therapist empathizes with their complicated feelings and inner anguish.

Case Example

Dr. Kenton was a 39-year-old critical care specialist whose chief complaint was "I recently learned that I am HIV positive. It's tougher than I thought." He was married and the father of two adolescent sons. He and his wife had not been sexually intimate with each other in many years. She was not infected. Dr. Kenton told his wife that he thought he had acquired the virus by a needle stick injury at work.

Becoming HIV positive did not come as a surprise to Dr. Kenton. He described himself as gay for as long as he could remember. His marriage was arranged by both families. "I love my wife. She is beautiful. She is kind. She is a phenomenal wife and mother. She adores me. And this is why being HIV positive is so hard for me. It is so unfair for her to have me sick like this, to live with the stigma of this disease. I have betrayed her and dishonored her. I am so guilty and so ashamed for my actions. I deserve this infection. I put myself at risk. I'm not afraid of dying. Dying would release me from my sin. My soul is tortured. It has been all my life because my religion does not accept homosexuality. I pray to God, 'why did you create me this way?' But my impulses never go away."

Separation and coming out as a gay man were anathema to Dr. Kenton. "In my culture you do not abandon your family. That is self-serving. As a man, as a husband and father, I am there for life. I am there to protect and provide. I have done that well, I believe. I am revered in my religious community as a physician, as a mentor and muse to young people. But you can imagine, can't you, how fraudulent I feel inside? If they knew how much I sin, I would have to die. But not by suicide, that is forbidden. I would slowly die of my self-hate and disgust. I would stop eating and hope for immune suppression and massive infection. Or dehydration."

This sad story illustrates how much one's religion and culture creates clinical symptoms and informs treatment. Some physicians coming of age at the same time as this man would have accepted their homosexuality and not married, or if they had married, they might have divorced and pursued life as a gay man. Furtive gay sex, always risky, was one of the few sexual options for this man. Although one might well assume that he would be afraid of a life-threatening disease, the truth is just the opposite. He feels he is deserving of punishment for his sinful transgression. His worry is for his wife, not himself. Therapy with this physician required much support and acceptance. Respecting his cultural and religious values was as pivotal as monitoring and treating his T cells, viral load, mood, and compulsive sexual behavior.

International Medical Graduates

International medical graduates make up approximately 25% of physicians in the U.S. medical workforce (Mullan 2005). They are a heterogeneous group of physicians who come from vastly different cultural, linguistic, and medical education backgrounds than their American colleagues (Rao et al. 2007). It has been estimated that 41% are from Asia, 12% from Pakistan, and 9% from the Philippines (Kramer 2006). Over half of IMGs in graduate medical education are either citizens or lawful immigrants from Caribbean island medical schools, such as St. George's in Grenada or Ross in Dominica (Brotherton et al. 2002). Demographic trends show that increasing numbers of IMGs are pursuing residencies in primary care specialties, internal medicine, and pediatrics (Brotherton et al. 2005).

There is little research on the mental health of IMGs. However, it is important to delineate some of the common challenges for IMGs—challenges that exist on top of the "normal" trials that all residents have as they pursue graduate medical education. These include becoming acculturated to North America; learning English, especially idioms and slang (if they are from non–English speaking countries); facing temporary periods of isolation from their peers; coping with a sense of longing for family and friends; preparing for one or more examinations; coming to terms with examination failure on first attempts; facing financial hurdles; confronting myriad medical licensing board regulations; facing discrimination; dealing with the stigma associated with emotional strain or psychiatric illness; and balancing the adoption of the values of North America with the preservation and abandonment of some of their home customs. Each of these challenges is no easy feat, and in the aggregate, the journey can become overwhelming.

Case Example

Dr. Mirwan, a fellow in endocrinology, called with this chief complaint: "I think I'm starting to behave a little weird at work." He was 33 years old, unmarried, and the only member of his family living abroad. Born in the Middle East, he came to North America to do residency training. Struggling with early morning wakening, crying outbursts, lowered self-esteem, poor appetite, and a 10-pound weight loss, he wondered if he was depressed. Then he added, "Or I wonder if I have a histrionic personality disorder." His psychiatrist confirmed the former and challenged the latter.

Statements from several interviews with Dr. Mirwan illustrated many of the strains contributing to his mood disorder. "Three members of my family are very ill. One is my brother—he's been diagnosed with multiple sclerosis. He doesn't deserve it." "I feel like I have failed them; if I were there I could oversee their care." "I am very closed, I don't talk about my feelings, I don't want to show my insecurities—and my culture is macho." "I have become too focused into myself, very self-absorbed—this is not good, not normal where I come from. That's why I worry that I have developed histrionic personality disorder since coming here." "I miss the intimacy of the Middle East; you people are different—cool, busy, no time to talk about things outside of medicine."

There was a family history of depression and suicide. The fact that Dr. Mirwan acknowledged this history was instrumental in his accepting the notion of antidepressant medication. He responded nicely to a selective serotonin uptake inhibitor and was compliant in taking it. Stigma was ever present, both at the beginning and during the entire time that he was in treatment: "I accept the biomedical part of depression, that I am genetically predisposed—as I am for diabetes—and that my neurotransmitters are off. But I am ashamed that I have depression. I feel deficient, not just chemically, but in strength and resistance to stress. As an IMG

I must be very guarded that no one learns of this. I am almost paranoid that if anyone in authority finds out, I will be asked to leave the residency and be deported home. I am made to feel 'lucky' to have this residency position. I must be very careful. Even though I know that mental illness exists globally, I believe also that I have shamed my home country by getting sick here. That geopolitically I have let her down. That as a visitor here, I must be a good ambassador."

The example of Dr. Mirwan illustrates some of the not uncommon stressors on IMGs. His depression has some psychosocial determinants that are important to uncover and work through in therapy. His words also highlight an added level of stigma in IMG physicians that aggravates the institutional stigma so commonly seen in physicians who develop symptoms of a psychiatric illness. An accepting and empathic approach by mental health professionals who treat IMGs helps tremendously in their efforts to regain self-worth and integrity. All "newcomers" struggle with feeling accepted and a sense of belonging, and IMGs are no exception.

What follows is an example of an IMG struggling with marital and family issues. This physician is also at a different professional and individual life stage than Dr. Mirwan. Her words and those of her husband are important to understand in the context of her ethnicity and culture. As psychiatrists, we are given the opportunity to learn so much about how all of us are shaped by both our family of origin and our country of origin, including the impact of acculturation on the next generation.

Case Example[1]

Dr. Vishnay, an obstetrician, complained that her husband, a businessman, seemed withdrawn and less involved in family life. Like her, he worked very long hours, but unlike her, he was frequently away on overseas trips. When he was home, he liked to play golf and spend time on his computer. She wondered if he was depressed or maybe having an affair. She thought he should be spending more time with their teenage sons.

In their psychiatrist's initial visit with the two of them, he learned that Dr. Vishnay had graduated from medical school in India. Her husband was at the same university studying commerce. They married shortly before coming to North America. She began her residency, and he completed his Master's degree in Business Administration. They started their family toward the end of her residency. They had a series of nannies when the boys were young and hired a housekeeper once they were both in school fulltime. Both Dr. and Mr. Vishnay were very successful in their careers. They lived in a beautiful home, their sons attended an elite private school, and they traveled at least twice a year to India to visit their families.

---

[1]Reprinted from Myers 2005 with permission of *Physician's Money Digest.*

When asked about his wife's concerns, Mr. Vishnay replied, "No I'm not depressed and I'm not having an affair. But I have pulled away from my wife. Why? She's obsessed with our sons becoming doctors. There is no other profession that meets her standards. She is very narrow in her thinking. She seems to respect what I do, yet when Sanjay talks about pursuing a business career she shuts him down. I feel insulted. You would think he wanted to be a tattoo artist by the expression of disgust on her face." Dr. Vishnay explained herself. "Medicine gives you autonomy, even in today's world of healthcare. Most people still respect physicians. I want our boys to be looked up to as children of immigrants, that not only did their parents succeed here but their children did too. Also it's very gratifying being a doctor and helping people."

Mr. Vishnay responded harshly: "Dare I say something that will embarrass you? I will. You are living vicariously through our sons. You want to brag about them to your colleagues. That they are on the honor roll and want to be *doctors*. Neither one has ever expressed an interest in medical school. You are programming them. And dare I say something else? I've never thought they were interested in health problems or in wanting to help people. They are both quite indulged, love expensive things, and just want to make a lot of money. Would you disagree?"

What transpired in this visit and a single follow-up visit was interesting. The subtext to Dr. Vishnay's goals for her sons was anxiety. She worried that she had neglected her children by having paid help. She loved being an obstetrician but felt guilty that she loved it too much. Even though she was raised by servants herself and had a good relationship with her mother, she felt insecure as a parent. She associated their following in her path as validation that she was a good mother.

The two of them agreed to change their interaction. Dr. Vishnay backed off and let her sons discover their own talents and aspirations, and her husband came forward and began spending time again with his sons.

In this example, we can learn a lot about the confluence of individual, dyadic, familial, and cultural values that underlie a chief complaint and its course. In many respects, Dr. Vishnay is no different than any other married, full-time female physician who is also a parent. She struggles with guilt—"Am I a good enough mother? Have I been home enough? Have I given too many hours, days, weeks to my work?"—and much like her married female physician colleagues, she worries about her husband's withdrawal. Is he having an affair? Is he depressed? However, what adds the unique cast here is an ethnic norm—being a doctor or lawyer is better than being another type of professional. Most of Dr. Vishnay's medical colleagues who are not IMGs or minority physicians would be delighted if their kids became a professional of any type. Dr. Vishnay seems to feel that she has failed as a working mother if her children do not follow her path, especially one that she enjoys so much.

Key Points

- Although there are some common personality traits in physicians, clinicians who treat minority and international medical graduate (IMG) physicians should always consider sociocultural customs and values that allow a more comprehensive biopsychosocial assessment and inform a broad-based treatment plan.

- Research on physicians who are members of minority and IMG groups is in its infancy. As we pursue continuing medical education and strive to improve our cultural competence on the front lines, we must keep an open mind and learn from our physician-patients and their families.

- Discrimination and stigma—both perceived and felt—are described by many minority and IMG physician-patients. These themes must be explored in the context of the doctor–patient relationship and fought vigorously in the context of the culture of medicine. Advocacy can be very effective in our training programs and wherever physicians work.

- Most minority and IMG physicians will be treated by someone outside of their reference group. State-of-the-art treatment is grounded in basic principles of acceptance, respect, and kindness. With these in place, healing can begin.

Psychiatric Evaluation of Physicians

The last thing most physicians want to be is a patient. They prefer to deny their vulnerability to illness and concentrate on the diseases of their patients. In this regard, the task of convincing the doctor to sit in the patient's chair in another physician's office may be a formidable challenge. This reluctance to seek help may vary somewhat by gender. In a recent review of the Colorado Physician Health Program physician client data from 1986 to 2006 (Gunderson 2006), the results indicated that male physicians are usually required to come for evaluation, but most female doctors present voluntarily. Nevertheless, the first step in helping a physician—that is, getting the doctor in the patient role—may require considerable resourcefulness.

Barriers to Care

There is a long historical legacy of physicians who continue to practice while impaired, sometimes causing harm to patients. Strong psychological resistances to seeking treatment are present within physicians, but there are also a number of systemic realities that reinforce these resistances. Finally, if physicians do find their way to a psychiatrist or other mental health professional, they often encounter obstacles and difficulties in receiving the same quality of care that others obtain. Each of these factors is considered separately here, but the barriers to good treatment for physicians are multifaceted and multidetermined, so there are times when all three of these factors converge.

Psychological Resistances

Many physicians live with internalized stigma about illness. Being ill makes them feel ashamed and disgraced. Although some physicians feel that any illness is stigmatizing, psychiatric illness in particular may be regarded with embarrassment. Physicians may blame themselves for becoming ill and fear that others will see them as weak or dependent. Physicians are often rugged individualists who use a classic triad of defenses to avoid facing illness in themselves— denial ("it's a simple cold, not pneumonia"), rationalization ("Of course I yell a lot at my kids; I'm a transplant surgeon, and my work is extremely stressful"), and minimization ("I only had two small drinks, honest, the Breathalyzer is wrong"). Moreover, for many physicians, overwork is the norm. They insist they are far too busy to see a doctor and too tired to eat properly and exercise. Physicians often will confess that they are terrified of what their symptoms might mean, so they refuse to go to a doctor for fear that he or she will confirm their worst fears and diagnose them with a dreaded disease. The patient role is foreign and demeaning to most physicians. They also hate to forfeit control and turn that control over to another physician.

Some physicians are better at self-care than others. As noted previously, Frank et al. (1998) found that women doctors were somewhat better than women in the general population at practicing preventive health measures. No such study of male physicians has been conducted. However, even doctors who are reasonably good about self-care may balk when needing to see a physician. Gendel (2005) pointed out that self-care does not require coping with the specter of actual illness. He noted: "Self-care activities also do not require a helper or treating physician (i.e., they do not require the physician to become a patient). Actual sickness and patienthood are not easy for physicians" (p. 50).

Systemic Barriers

Stigma about illness does not reside only in the psyche of the individual physician. It is magnified as it expands to the house of medicine as a whole. When the entire profession collectively insists on a denial of self-care and a stigmatization of illness as weakness, it reinforces denial of symptoms and delayed recognition of the need for help in case of the individual doctor. Extremely ill physicians may eschew treatment altogether, and this decision aggravates morbidity and increases mortality, especially death by suicide. Stigma may be accurately perceived, as in an actual judgment by colleagues, or may be feared without objective verification, such as an inner sense that one will be judged. Exclusion clauses in disability insurance plans also present a barrier to care. Residents and medical students without comprehensive insurance coverage in place may be terrified to seek help because of this concern. Some physicians will avoid psychiatric care if they fear they will have to answer blanket questions and make detailed disclosures of confidential treatment when they apply for a medical license or when their current license is up for renewal. We return to this matter in detail later in this chapter. Computerized pharmacy networks in the physician's locale of practice may frighten the ill physician whose psychiatrist has written a prescription for medication. Some will self-medicate to avoid being identified in a pharmacy database. Indeed, self-medication and self-treatment are huge problems. For many physicians, there is no other form of healthcare. Finally, some families of physicians do not accept that their loved one has a mental illness and requires treatment. They may undermine much-needed care or reinforce the embarrassment and self-loathing that the doctor is already experiencing with their manner of relating to the physician. They may also worry that seeking treatment will result in loss of livelihood.

Barriers Deriving From the Quality of Treatment

Despite their commitment, training, and experience with psychiatric disorders, not all psychiatrists and mental health professionals have purged themselves of the internalized stigma that they incorporated while growing up in a society that has always viewed the mentally ill as different, inferior, weak, or violent. Thus treaters of physicians may have great difficulty in providing doctors with the same quality of care that they provide to others. Some psychiatrists will practice with a biomedical rigidity and thus avoid uncovering or treating psychosocial forces that underlie the emotional distress in the physician seeking help. Instead, they overly rely on medication while devaluing psychotherapy. This approach may alienate symptomatic physicians who desire more comprehensive treatment. In rural and underserved areas, psychiatrists may not be available to look after ill physicians. Physicians who are practicing in the community may find the relationship too close with the local psychiatrist(s) because they are colleagues or feel they have a conflict of interest. Finally, many psychiatrists have never educated themselves, either formally or informally, on the subject of physician health. They are thus not attuned to the special issues that make physicians somewhat unique as patients. Doctors who consult them often leave feeling disappointed, confused, or angry.

The Problem of Reporting

Another disconcerting historical trend has been reluctance on the part of colleagues to report an impaired physician or reach out to a colleague who is self-destructing.

Case Example

Dr. Wilson was a 29-year-old surgery resident who developed low back pain from standing at the operating table for long hours during his third postgraduate year of training. He began treating himself with oral codeine tablets that he had on hand from an oral surgery procedure. When he ran out, he prescribed more for his girlfriend, who then passed them on to him. He soon developed tolerance and kept escalating the dosage and the route of administration. Before long he was addicted to intravenous Demerol (meperidine) and periodically injected himself in the doctors' locker room prior to surgery in full view of colleagues, none of whom reported him. When his condition was finally revealed following an overdose, several colleagues acknowledged that they were aware of his addiction, but they did not want to ruin his career by reporting him.

The reluctance of colleagues to report Dr. Wilson reflects the long-standing concern that such behavior will be treated as a disciplinary matter rather than an illness in need of treatment. As early as 1975, the American Medical Association recognized this problem and developed model legislation to offer therapeutic alternatives for addicted physicians who faced board discipline (Andrews 2005). Physicians were much more likely to report themselves or colleagues if confidential treatment contracts were available.

Since the mid-1970s, the recognition that physicians have a hard time accepting illness and adhering to treatment has led to the development of physician health programs (PHPs) in almost all 50 states and almost all provinces in Canada. In the United States, most PHPs are sponsored by state medical societies. If a physician referred through a PHP complies with the rehabilitation program established by the PHP, no report is made to the licensing board. If the physician-patient does not comply or experiences a relapse of a serious illness like bipolar disorder or alcoholism, the case may be turned over to the licensing board. Most of these programs monitor other conditions in addition to chemical dependency, although addiction treatment has been the basic conceptual model of operation.

Although PHPs are usually separate from licensing boards, the interface of the two entities varies from state to state. In some states, only certain problematic behaviors can be excluded from the licensing board. If, for example, a physician has had sexual relationships with patients or poses a danger to self or others, reporting to the board may be mandated. Some licensing boards work more collaboratively than others and have diversion programs that refer physicians to PHPs that are actually run by the board itself. Some PHPs engage in monitoring of physicians, whereas others are limited to support and advocacy, because the board does all the monitoring. In 2001 the Joint Commission for the Accreditation of Healthcare Organizations established a requirement for hospitals to make available a process to address physician health issues separate from disciplinary proceedings.

Running throughout this dialectic between discipline and treatment or between concern for the public safety and concern for privacy is the complex distinction between being "ill" and "impaired." *Impairment* in physicians has many definitions, but what is cited most often is thus:

> Impairment should be defined as the inability of a licensee to practice medicine with reasonable skill and safety by reason of:
>
> - Mental illness;
> - Physical illness or condition, including, but not limited to, those illnesses or conditions that would adversely affect cognitive, motor or perceptual skills; or
> - Habitual or excessive use or abuse of drugs defined by law as controlled substances, or alcohol or of other substances that impair ability (Federation of State Medical Boards 2000, p. 26)

Mental illness in physicians is not synonymous with impairment (Myers 1996c). In fact, the vast majority of physicians who are in treatment with a mental health professional are not impaired. They are working and practicing medicine safely and competently, although they may be working at reduced capacity or curtailing the full range of their services until they are well. They are accepting treatment voluntarily, and their identities and illnesses are unknown to their state or provincial licensing board, employers, and colleagues.

Similarly, addiction does not automatically imply impairment. Actual impairment of work functioning generally does not appear until late in the course of addictive disease (Gendel 2006). Lack of knowledge or skill necessary to practice medicine also is not impairment; this problem should more appropriately be regarded as incompetence.

How big a problem is impairment? An estimated 7%–12% of practicing physicians become impaired at some point. Of these physicians, 75% have chemical dependency (discussed in Chapter 5, "Addictions: Chemical and Nonchemical"), 6%–20% have a psychiatric illness, and the remainder have cognitive impairment associated with brain disease such as dementia or other physical illnesses. The most common impairing conditions are substance abuse and dependence, mood disorders (especially major depressive disorder and bipolar affective disorder, types 1 and 2), concurrent or comorbid conditions (anxiety and mood disorders plus substance abuse and dependence), delusional disorders, organic disorders, and eating disorders (severe with malnutrition and behavioral disturbances).

It is wise to remember that unrelenting situational crises—intense marital and financial stress, burnout, chronic overwork, and fatigue—can cause sufficient distraction, preoccupation, and weariness to be classified as physician impairment (Walzer 1990).

Physicians can be quite symptomatic and not be impaired. Impairment is not always static or absolute; hence, physician-patients may be impaired at times and not others. Or the physician may be impaired in some medical settings and not others. Impairment in the physician health field usually refers to occupational impairment. Spouses may describe their husband or wife as very impaired at home in the evenings and on weekends because of heavy alcohol intake, but this description does not necessarily mean that they are unable to practice medicine safely and competently during the workday or work week. Some state licensing boards have glossed over the distinction between "ill" and "impaired" and make it difficult for physicians to seek treatment because of fear that the licensing board will stigmatize them as "impaired." Applications to licensing boards may require physicians to reveal if they have ever had treatment for a psychiatric condition. In some cases, those who have been treated for depression have been required to undergo an expensive evaluation by a forensic psychiatrist.

Physicians in the state of Arkansas successfully argued that asking license applicants such questions needlessly stigmatized doctors who had psychiatric disorders and discouraged them from seeking help (Moran 2006). They were able to change the language on the application for a medical license so the psychiatric conditions were not singled out. Moreover, they made a major change in physician privacy by specifying that only those treatments that were *required* by a licensing, credentialing, or privileging body had to be reported. Prior to these changes, all treatments for psychiatric disorders had to be reported, resulting in major ramifications for employment, let alone individual emotional turmoil. The physicians had to either lie and risk a felony charge or face bureaucratic barriers and violation of their privacy. In some states today, like Colorado, one can answer "no" to questions about psychiatric disorders or substance abuse on an application for licensure or re-licensure if the physician's condition is known to the PHP of the state.

Other encroachments on privacy also may occur. Some licensing boards require that the ongoing treatment of the physician identified as having a mental disorder cannot be conducted under the usual confines of doctor–patient confidentiality. The treating physician may have to make regular reports to the licensing board about the physician-patient, thus compromising the confidentiality of psychiatric treatment.

In any case, it behooves physicians or other clinicians who evaluate and treat doctors to know the reporting requirements in their state or province.

Serving Both the Patient and the Public

An underlying theme in these concerns about privacy and reporting involves the fact that professionals who treat colleagues have a dual responsibility—good

TABLE 3–1.   Sources of referral

- Licensing board
- Physician health program
- Risk management committee of a hospital
- Dean, department chair, or training director
- Attorney in the context of pending litigation
- Colleagues in a group practice
- Primary care physician
- Psychotherapist
- Family or friend
- Self-referral

psychiatric care of the physician-patient and protection of the public from an impaired practitioner. Hence psychiatrists and other mental health professionals involved in a physician evaluation may feel like "double agents." They cannot limit themselves to a traditional helping role that places the patient's needs first. They must balance that role with another ethical concern—the public good.

The sources of referral outlined in Table 3–1 indicate that in many cases the dual function derives from the origin of the request for the evaluation. Some of these agencies requesting referral may pay for the evaluation, whereas others will expect the physician to pay for his or her own evaluation. Regardless of the responsibility for payment, however, all will expect a report of the findings and recommendations stemming from the evaluation. Hence the evaluating clinician must obtain a signed release of information at the beginning of the evaluation so that it is understood by the physician being evaluated that the process is not confidential. For clinical, legal, and ethical reasons, the physician who is in the patient role should also be sent a copy of the report that is going to the licensing board, PHP, or other organization. If the physician-patient refuses to sign a release or wishes to see the final report before authorizing the disclosure to the referral source, the evaluating clinician must explain to the physician that withholding the release may be self-defeating in that it will have adverse effects with the referral source. For example, if the PHP cannot receive a report, it may choose not to advocate for the patient. A hospital risk management committee may simply suspend the privileges of a physician who refuses to have the report sent as part of the evaluation.

In the United States the Health Insurance Portability and Accountability Act of 1996 (HIPAA) added some legal "teeth" to the evaluator's insistence on a release before starting the evaluation. As required by HIPAA, the Department of Health and Human Services adopted the privacy rule, which explicitly states that a signed release to the third party requesting the independent medical evaluation is a condition of performing the evaluation (Gold and Metzner 2006). Insistence on a signed release is also protective of the evaluator. Legal immunity is frequently not available for these evaluations that determine impairment. Moreover, the record needs to be written with the assumption that the evaluee may ultimately obtain it and use it as a legal document. Gold and Metzner (2006) recommended that five key issues should be discussed at the beginning of an evaluation:

- The identity of the referral source
- The understanding of both evaluator and evaluee of the reason for the referral
- The potential consequences of the assessment
- Who will ultimately receive a copy of the evaluator's report
- The evaluee's understanding of his or her access to the report

One should also clarify that even though the assessment may be helpful to the physician, the major purpose is to evaluate rather than help.

Although the concept of the therapeutic alliance does not apply in its usual sense to the setting of an evaluation mandated by a third party, the evaluating clinician might think in terms of an *evaluation alliance* when approaching the patient. While fully recognizing the "double agency" involved in the process, the evaluating clinician can also encourage the physician to see such an assessment as an opportunity for self-reflection and self-knowledge. Even if the evaluation is required, the physician-patient may use it to his or her advantage to learn more about the stresses inherent in the practice of medicine, psychological characteristics that may exacerbate those stressors, and the nature of the practice setting itself that are problematic. Moreover, the evaluating clinician can clarify again and again that one of the main purposes of the evaluation is to see if it is possible to identify optimal treatment strategies that may help the physician-patient in the long run.

When physicians first come to a psychiatric evaluation, they often feel victimized by their colleagues, their risk management committee, the licensing board, or other agencies. Sometimes the manner in which they are told of complaints about them can make them feel that others are "ganging up" on them. A frequent refrain one hears is something like, "There are many other physicians in my hospital who are much worse than I am. I have no idea why I got picked for an evaluation. They need it worse than I do." Often the physicians in such situations will assert that they are pawns in a complex political matrix within the hospital or clinic where they work. In some cases, this characterization may be true. They also may be convinced that the complaints against them are false or totally overblown. Many argue that they have not been given a chance to explain themselves. They may come to an evaluation seeking vindication. Clinicians who are conducting the evaluation may need to explain to the physician-patient that the goal of an evaluation is rather modest. The evaluating team will determine if there are emotional problems, if they are treatable in a reasonable treatment or rehabilitation program, and whether or not it is safe for the physician-patient to practice medicine. The evaluation is not a court of law where one's guilt or innocence can be established, and the politics of any healthcare system are far beyond the scope of what mental health professionals in the evaluation setting can tackle.

The Structure of the Evaluation

An evaluation usually begins with a phone call from the referring body or, if it is a situation of self-referral, from the physician himself or herself. Sometimes another mental health professional refers a patient because of concerns about diagnosis and treatment. In any case, during this initial conversation the evaluating clinician must obtain a detailed account of the circumstances leading to the evaluation. Several questions need to be addressed:

- What are the charges or complaints against the physician?
- Is this part of a longstanding pattern or an incident that is entirely out of character for the physician?
- Are there previous complaints against the physician in a personnel file or the licensing board record?
- Is the physician's competence or ability to safely practice medicine in question?
- Have there been observations that lead one to suspect alcohol or drug abuse?
- Do the complaints come from patients, coworkers, colleagues, or all of the above?
- Has the physician been told about the concerns, and if so, what was his or her reaction?
- Has the physician been placed on leave from a hospital or has there been action on the physician's license by the licensing board?

After a thorough discussion of the reasons for referral, it is useful to have the referred physician call the evaluating clinician so they can get to know each other a bit over the telephone and so that the clinician can hear the physician's perspective on the nature of the concerns or complaints. Many times, the physician will view the evaluator as an extension of the body that made the referral and question the clinician's objectivity. It may be helpful to stress in the initial con-

tact that the evaluation is being done independently without preconceived notions about whose account is accurate. Matters such as who sees the final report
and the method of payment are also taken up from the initial contact.

Collateral information must be a high priority. The referral source should
send copies of all complaints or concerns in the physician's file. The physician-
patient must arrange for records of previous treatment to be sent to the evaluating
team as well as any previous psychological testing or other relevant records. An
evaluation may have little merit if it is confined solely to the verbal report of the
physician-patient. A basic fact of human nature is that we never see ourselves as
others do. We are all masters at self-deception, and an outside perspective is of
great value in assessing problematic behaviors. When we see ourselves on videotape, we often react by saying, "That's not me! I don't look that way or sound that
way!" We are often shocked at the way others regard us. This information is crucial
for helping physicians understand how they come across to others. In this regard,
including the physician's spouse, partner, or other family member in the evaluation process may be critically important in getting the full picture.

Case Example

Dr. Jenkins was a hospitalist who was thought by all of his colleagues and coworkers to be an outstanding physician. His patients felt they received good care
from him, and he had had no patient complaints in his 20-year practice. However, he had accumulated quite a file of written concerns from fellow physicians
and from nurses and other healthcare staff at his hospital. The major focus of
the concerns was that he came across as angry, intimidating, and menacing. The
people with whom he worked were afraid of him, but they did not want to say
anything to him because they feared his response. When the president of the
medical staff and the hospital chief executive officer suggested he seek evaluation, Dr. Jenkins was horrified. He insisted that no one found him intimidating
and that he was easy to get along with.

At the time he came for his assessment, he told the evaluating psychiatrist
that the hospital staff liked working with him and had told him so. He admitted
to having something of a "hot temper," but he insisted that it was not anything
serious and he always got over his anger quickly. He also said that he apologized
to anyone who was a target of his anger. His wife, who sat in on the initial session
of the evaluation, said to Dr. Jenkins, "Honey, you don't understand how intimidating you are. You're six-three, and you lumber around the hospital in a way
that makes people think you might run them over." She went on to say that their
15-year-old son was terrified of his dad and was afraid to show him his grades if
they were anything less than perfect. Dr. Jenkins was shocked to hear that his son
feared him that way, and he had great difficulty hearing what his wife had to say.
The evaluation involved a gradual acceptance that the perspective of others was
different from his own and that there was legitimacy to that perspective.

The case of Dr. Jenkins illustrates the value of collateral information. When
the spouse or partner cannot travel because of child care or work responsibili-

ties or expense, a phone interview is often extraordinarily rewarding in gaining this additional information. Parents or children of the physician can be equally useful as observers of the physician's personality style.

Communication with the referral source is of great importance in conducting an evaluation. From the initial contact onward, the evaluating professional must have a clear idea of the questions the referral source wishes to be answered in the course of an evaluation. Sometimes those questions cannot be clearly articulated, and the referral source may need help in spelling them out. In some cases, there is a secret wish that the evaluating clinician will find a way to get rid of the doctor so the hospital, clinic, or other organization does not have to do the difficult and painful work of letting someone go. The evaluating clinician needs to clarify that an assessment of emotional problems is not the same thing as adjudicating the most appropriate discipline for the physician-patient. Although the two things may be related, they are separately assigned. A hospital risk management committee may refer to a licensing board or a medical staff committee to think through appropriate discipline but will want an independent evaluation of psychiatric status from an outside clinician.

The reasons for referral are highly varied and are summarized in Table 3–2. Some of these categories, such as irresponsible behavior involving recordkeeping, are more likely to come from institutions where physicians work, whereas others, such as marital problems, may involve a spouse or partner who drags the physician to a professional for help in convincing him or her that a problem exists. Still others, such as depression or burnout, may be brought to light by observations of colleagues who see that the physician is "just not like himself." The description of the problems, whatever they may be, must be reasonably comprehensive before the evaluation begins.

On the basis of the advance information received by the clinician who heads up the evaluation process, a number of different components can be added to the assessment. In some cases, one psychiatrist or other mental health professional does everything by himself or herself. Another model is a team evaluation that takes place over a few days, on either an inpatient or an outpatient basis, where several different evaluators from various disciplines collaborate in a multidisciplinary assessment. For example, a psychiatrist may do individual psychiatric interviews, a psychologist may conduct an extensive battery of psychological tests, and a social worker may do family assessment as part of the process. Other components that one might wish to include in cases of suspected substance abuse are urine drug screenings as well as blood work that may reflect relevant physiological changes. A complete medical evaluation is usually indicated as well, although often that may be done separately in advance of the psychiatric evaluation. When there are specific problem areas that require special expertise, consultants can be involved if needed. For example, in the following case, both a chemical dependency expert and a bipolar expert supplemented psychiatric in-

TABLE 3–2. Common reasons for referral

- Chemical dependency
- Disruptive behavior
- Poor anger management
- Irresponsibility in the workplace: documentation and timeliness of records, responding to pages
- Defiance of authority
- Depression or burnout
- Prescribing problems
- Concerns about clinical judgment
- Bizarre or psychotic behavior
- Dementia or other cognitive dysfunction
- Suicidal behavior
- Financial problems or questionable billing practices
- Sexual harassment
- Sexual misconduct with patients
- Nonsexual boundary violations
- Marital problems

terviews by the team leader psychiatrist and an advanced psychiatric resident. The example illustrates how a multidisciplinary assessment team works together and reaches final conclusions involving diagnosis and treatment recommendations.[1]

Case Example

Dr. Allen was a 36-year-old married male internist who was referred for a comprehensive diagnostic assessment from his state's physician health program. The referring physicians had concerns about diagnostic issues, particularly if there was a personality disorder or a mood disorder in addition to known substance abuse and also whether a treatment and rehabilitation plan might be helpful in Dr. Allen's case. Dr. Allen had already surrendered his medical license because of chemical dependency.

---

[1]This case was published in different form in the *American Journal of Psychiatry* Clinical Case Conference series (Petersen-Crair et al. 2003).

Dr. Allen was interviewed by the psychiatrist who headed the evaluation team and the chief resident of the clinic where the assessment took place. He was also interviewed by a bipolar expert as a consultant and an addictions expert as a second consultant. He underwent an extensive battery of psychological tests administered by two psychologists, and the team had advance records so that his history was well established.

Dr. Allen had had mood symptoms since childhood. He was diagnosed with depression when he was a first-year medical student and was offered samples of fluoxetine. He was later treated with nefazodone, which he discontinued on his own. Prior to coming for the evaluation, he had been prescribing venlafaxine for himself. He developed symptoms of hypomania when the dosage of venlafaxine was increased to 300 mg/day, but he had had no previous history of clear episodes of mania.

Dr. Allen had started drinking heavily at age 17 and continued heavy drinking throughout college and medical school. By the time he was a resident, his drinking had escalated to the point where he was intoxicated most weekends when he was not on call or moonlighting. He had entered a residential rehabilitation program, which led to approximately 3 years of abstinence from alcohol. After his completion of residency, he went into solo practice and began to prescribe himself tramadol when he developed tension headaches. He gradually increased the dosage of tramadol to about 1.25–2.5 g/day. He remained abstinent from alcohol and attended Alcoholics Anonymous (AA) meetings regularly. As he increased the dosage of tramadol, however, he experienced euphoria, and he felt he no longer needed to attend AA meetings. Eventually he increased the dosage of tramadol to an average of 5–6 g/day. On one occasion it induced a grand mal seizure while he was performing a minor medical procedure.

After moving to a new state to start a new practice, he began drinking heavily and was spending up to $1,000 a month to sustain his tramadol habit. He worked long hours with an erratic sleep schedule and started experiencing marital stress because he was never home. He said his wife would yell and scream at him, and he felt he was reexperiencing the violence of his childhood. She had threatened divorce, and he again entered a rehabilitation program. While in a halfway house associated with the program, he became involved in a physical altercation with one of the other patients there and was hauled off by the police. He also made sexual overtures to a female patient there. He was then discharged from the halfway house.

Dr. Allen's developmental history was replete with trauma. He had witnessed his mother having sex with a number of different lovers while his father was on the road as a truck driver. He had also witnessed extreme violence between his mother and her lovers. The trauma escalated until he had to be removed from his mother's household by Social Services. His father was an alcoholic, and there was an extensive history of alcoholism throughout his family. He married at an early age and had had a stormy relationship throughout his marriage. He repeatedly engaged in verbal arguments and occasionally had physical altercations with his wife. Many of his relapses occurred after these fights. He and his wife did not seek consistent marital therapy, and they were separated at the time of the evaluation, so his wife did not want to participate. Dr. Allen acknowledged that he feared abandonment and realized that he might unintentionally drive away women before they abandon him first.

At the time of his evaluation, he was taking venlafaxine (sustained release) 225 mg/day, divalproex 500 mg bid, and doxepin, 75 mg/day. He had not taken tramadol for approximately 4 months at the time of his evaluation.

A mental status examination revealed that Dr. Allen was a casually dressed, moderately obese man who appeared his stated age. He was oriented to place, person, time, and situation. He was cooperative and polite throughout the evaluation. He had good eye contact and revealed no motoric abnormalities. His thought processes were well organized but slightly slowed and somewhat over-inclusive in the number of details he provided. He showed no evidence of a thought disorder or flight of ideas, and his mood appeared euthymic. He denied suicidal ideation. His affect was constricted, with only rare expressions of emotion.

The neuropsychologists on the team were asked to evaluate the patient for potential cognitive impairments that may result from chronic alcohol and substance abuse and to establish whether he could function mentally at a level commensurate with the complexities of medical practice. In addition, the presence of serious character pathology needed to be assessed, along with the possibility of bipolar illness. The psychologists used the Wechsler Adult Intelligence Scale–II (Wechsler 1997), the California Verbal Learning Test (Delis et al. 2000), Trail Making Tests A and B (Partington and Leiter 1979), the Stroop Color-Word Interference Test (Golden 1976), the Controlled Oral Word Association Test (Spreen and Benton 1977), and the Hooper Visuospatial Organizational Test (Hooper 1958). In addition, projective testing with the Rorschach (Khadivi et al. 1997), the Thematic Apperception Test, and the Incomplete Sentence Test (Rotter 1950) was carried out. The Minnesota Multiphasic Personality Inventory–2 and the Personality Assessment Inventory scales (Morley 1991) suggested significant affective instability. Dr. Allen was found to score higher on his verbal skills than on his nonverbal skills. Marked differences of this kind are known concomitants of chronic alcohol and drug abuse. His memory was unimpaired, as was his executive cognitive functioning. Overall, the test findings suggested comorbid Axis I and Axis II pathology and a complex clinical syndrome necessitating a guarded prognosis.

The consultant with expertise in bipolar affective disorder noted that Dr. Allen described episodes that were phenomenologically consistent with hypomania, including increased speech, flight of ideas, increased energy, and increased confidence. These episodes lasted no more than several days at a time and appeared to be isolated to times when he was either abusing prescription drugs and/or taking antidepressants. She noted that the current nomenclature indicates that hypomanic periods occurring only in the context of antidepressant treatment are not considered bipolar disorder. These patients would be considered to have a bipolar spectrum disorder and are still treated with mood stabilizers on the basis of extrapolation from data on the treatment of bipolar depression.

The chemical dependency consultant, also a psychiatrist, noted the extensive family history of alcoholism and the patient's tendency to self-prescribe drugs such as tramadol to the point of seizure induction. He felt that Dr. Allen satisfied the traditional definition of an impaired physician and that he was unable to practice medicine with reasonable skill and safety to patients because of excessive use or abuse of drugs and alcohol (Parsons and Farr 1981). He felt the most accurate diagnosis from the substance abuse standpoint would be polysubstance dependence.

He noted that Dr. Allen was still relapsing regularly despite recovery and rehabilitation efforts.

All of the evaluators sat down for a meeting to synthesize their data. All agreed that Dr. Allen had a picture of complex comorbidity. Indeed, although the term "impaired physician" often is associated with chemical dependency, detailed evaluation frequently reveals more complex psychopathology. A biopsychosocial perspective was necessary for a thorough understanding of the patient. Biological factors, such as genetic contributions to the mood disorder and alcoholism, interacted with environmental trauma from childhood to produce the clinical picture. Dr. Allen had a bipolar spectrum disorder in addition to the polysubstance abuse and also had signs of Cluster B personality disorder even while sober and euthymic. These personality disorder features included impulsivity, poor judgment, problematic interpersonal relationships, and identity diffusion. He had gotten into fights, approached women with sexual intent in a highly inappropriate manner, and had difficulty integrating his personal role with his professional behavior. Despite his complex comorbid conditions, Dr. Allen was viewed as deeply devoted to the practice of medicine. The team wondered if his zeal to treat others and heal them might be partially determined by an unsuccessful effort to cure his mother of her suffering when he was a child. The trauma he had experienced in his childhood had taken its toll. He grew up with a fragmented self so that a dedicated physician coexisted side-by-side with an aspect of himself that was impulsive, irresponsible, and self-destructive. The two remained unintegrated and caused him great difficulty in understanding himself. The team then outlined an optimal treatment and rehabilitation plan:

1. Attend three AA meetings per week and continue working with his sponsor.
2. Have at least twice-weekly urine drug screens.
3. Continue treatment in his halfway house for the time being.
4. Seek weekly marital therapy (with his wife), because many of the triggers that cause him to use substances were related to marital issues.
5. Establish himself with a primary care doctor who prescribes his medication.
6. Do no self-prescribing whatsoever.
7. See a psychiatrist on a regular basis to prescribe mood stabilizers. The team suggested moving his divalproex to bedtime and tapering his doxepin. Trials of lithium and perhaps lamotrigine were also recommended.
8. Consider long-term individual dynamically oriented therapy. The team felt that long-term individual dynamically oriented therapy might help him to deal with his traumatic childhood and focus on integrating the fragments of his self into a more coherent identity. Therapy would also help him to anticipate the consequences of his actions, increase his capacity to understand how others' internal worlds are different from his own, and process feelings without using substances.

The team saw Dr. Allen as incapable of safely practicing medicine at the time of the evaluation and suggested that he embark on a comprehensive rehabilitation program and not consider working in medicine again until he had maintained sobriety for 12 months and was well launched in his other treatments. If the rehabilitation plan went smoothly and he remained free from relapse, it was recommended that he might be able to work in an institutional setting under careful supervision. It was also recommended that he should keep regular hours so that his sleep cycle was not disrupted. Finally, the team recommended that he continue monitoring under the auspices of the state physicians' health program.

The case of Dr. Allen may be more complicated than that of most physicians who are seen by an evaluation team for the first time. Nevertheless, comorbid conditions are frequently present and missed if a thorough evaluation is not conducted.

Dr. Allen was readily accepting of his diagnoses and treatment plan because he had recognized his difficulties prior to the evaluation. Many other physicians are in a state of denial and deeply resist the idea that their problems are worse than their colleagues' and thus require some form of monitoring or treatment. Considerable tact and persuasiveness may be necessary at the time of evaluation to convince the physician that the problems are real and must be addressed. Sometimes only the threat of action on the physician's license or suspension from a medical staff may motivate the physician to comply with treatment. Some will only go through the motions of treatment and thus need to "bottom out" before their motivation is genuine. In such cases, additional forms of monitoring, such as contact with collateral sources and face-to-face interviews, may be needed (Gendel 2006). A substantial number, however, are accepting of the help and feel relief that their problems have finally been recognized and are viewed as treatable and manageable.

When patients are particularly resistant to hearing the diagnostic findings, the psychological testing can be a valuable aid to the evaluating clinician. For example, in the case of Dr. Allen, the team was able to document a disparity between verbal and nonverbal IQ scores, suggesting the effect of long-term substance abuse on the patient's brain. This finding was highly disconcerting to Dr. Allen and led him to increase his resolve to be abstinent. Similarly, when disturbing personality traits are present, the physician-patient may disavow any validity to those traits when they are merely the clinical impressions of an interviewer. However, when these traits appear on testing, the evaluating team can say to the patient in many cases, "These are things that you said about yourself on the tests." Hence the testing may carry more weight with the patient in that the conclusions reached are based on the physician's own words, not simply the interviewer's impressions. However, some physician-patients will read up on the tests to "prep" themselves for the evaluation or to find ammunition to dispute the validity of the tests.

The here-and-now behavior of the physician-patient during the evaluation may be of extraordinary value. When, for example, there are disturbing interactions reported in the complaints about a physician, evaluators should keep in mind that the same kind of interpersonal behavior that occurs in the workplace is likely to appear in the course of the evaluation.

Case Example

Dr. Sanders was a 43-year-old endocrinologist who had had seven different complaints filed against him, all of which concerned sexual harassment. He had never directly approached a female coworker and asked her to have sexual relations; rather, the women complained that he made inappropriate jokes, looked at female coworkers in a certain way, and would touch his genitals in front of women. This set of behaviors created a hostile work environment for female employees, and several of them wanted to be transferred to areas where they would not encounter Dr. Sanders. The physician himself was flabbergasted to hear these complaints and denied that these descriptions were accurate.

When he underwent the evaluation, he arrived in a shirt whose collar was open far enough to reveal a pendant that he was wearing around his neck. He carried himself with a swagger and a demeanor suggesting a man who was overly confident with women. During the course of three different interviews with three different female doctors who were part of the evaluation team, he scratched his genitals in front of each of the evaluators numerous times during their interviews. This behavior made all three women uncomfortable, and they noted that he was oblivious to the impact the behavior had on them. When presenting the results of the findings to him, the evaluating team was able to point out that the things that happened in the workplace were repeating themselves in the interview and therefore provided a glimpse into the dynamics that occur with other women. Specifically, he was not consciously aware of how his behavior was impacting those around him.

The case of Dr. Sanders reflects a crucially important theme for evaluators: often problematic behaviors that bring a physician to an assessment have nothing to do with impairment. Rather, the behaviors reflect problems in professionalism. In recent years a good deal of attention has been given to this long-neglected aspect of physician behavior (Stern 2006; Stern and Papadakis 2006). Professionalism is now considered one of the core competencies in medical education, and a quiet revolution is going on throughout the field as behaviors that once were tolerated within the profession as long as the doctor was performing competently are no longer permissible. Such things as shouting or throwing instruments in the operating room, treating lower-paid hospital staff with contempt or verbal abuse, humiliating medical students, or publicly bad-mouthing colleagues are examples of lack of professionalism that many healthcare facilities tolerated for years because of a tradition within medicine of not challenging the physician.

Although the exact definition of *professionalism* is challenging because it involves so many different dimensions, a useful one is provided by Arnold and Stern (2006): "Professionalism is demonstrated through a foundation of clinical competence, communication skills, and ethical and legal understanding, upon which is built the aspiration to, and wise application of, the principles of professionalism: excellence, humanism, accountability, and altruism" (p. 19).

Fundamental to these principles of professionalism is the notion that the physician must behave in a way that exemplifies compassion and caring in every aspect of one's professional activities—including how one treats others in the workplace. The definition also suggests that a process of reflection is necessary to recognize the impact that one's words or actions have on others, whether patients or employees. Hence many evaluations will readily dispense with the issue of impairment, because the issue of competence to practice medicine is clear, but focus instead on professional behaviors that create problems for the physician and others in a work setting. These must be taken as seriously as concerns about impairment. More detailed discussion of problems of professionalism will be covered in Chapter 6 ("Personality Disorders, Personality Traits, and Disruptive Physicians").

This vignette about Dr. Sanders is emblematic of a frequent problem in providing the results of an evaluation to the physician-patient. Often the evaluator must deliver news that is not welcome or is even totally rejected. A climate must be created throughout the evaluation period in which the physician-patient feels understood, recognized, and empathically validated. At the time of the last meeting when the feedback from the evaluation is provided to the patient, the evaluators must be able to emphasize positive qualities as well as the problems that brought the physician-patient to attention. Hence it is well advised to begin with the strengths, such as intelligence, competence as a physician (if present), and the positive intentions of the physician to help others. When providing comments about major problem areas, the evaluators should also provide hope for remediation. Because many of the physician-patients feel overwhelmed with the information they are hearing verbally, some evaluators prefer to send a written report to the patient covering the same information. As noted earlier, the physician-patient should receive the same written report that is given to the referral source. With this in mind, psychiatric jargon and esoteric language should be kept to a minimum.

Special Situations

At times, the evaluators will conclude that the physician is too impaired to practice medicine and that no amount of treatment or rehabilitation is likely to remediate the problems. Examples include progressive dementia, terminal cancer, severe physical disability, antisocial characterological traits, repeated boundary violations, and refractory chemical dependency. In such situations, the evaluators must tactfully convey to the physician-patient that the practice of medicine must be given up. This news can be shattering to physicians who have their core identity inextricably tied to the idea of being a physician. It may be helpful to clarify the reasons for the recommendation and emphasize the idea that patient safety must be the paramount concern in such a decision. Sometimes, comments such as, "We know you have the patients' best interests at heart, and therefore we know that you would not want to keep practicing if patients are placed at risk," may be useful. It is ideal for a spouse or other family members to be present at the time that these conclusions are delivered so that they can serve as allies to the evaluating team and help the physician accept the inevitable. Some physicians can be encouraged to seek out employment in other areas if they are still cognitively and physically able. Others can be directed toward retirement planning opportunities so that they can continue to be productive in other areas of life. Above all, clinicians who are evaluating such physicians must not shirk the responsibility of making these tough decisions. They, too, must keep patient welfare paramount in their minds. If there is any concern that the physician could become suicidal, it is wise to contact the referral source in advance or after the meeting.

Another situation that may arise is that at the end of an extensive psychiatric evaluation, no emotional causes of impairment are found. Nevertheless, the evaluation team may be frankly uncertain regarding whether the physician is competent to practice. There may be concerns that the physician went to a medical school or residency that provided inferior training. There may be concerns that the physician's intelligence is simply not up to par to practice medicine competently. With elderly physicians, there may be concerns that a physician has not kept up with advances in medicine and should not be practicing with the limited fund of knowledge that he or she possesses. In these situations, the patient can be referred to programs around North America such as the Center for Personalized Education for Physicians (www.cpepdoc.org), which puts physicians through a series of tests designed to determine physician competence quite apart from physical or emotional impairment. By referring the physician to one of these programs, evaluating teams can take one more step in assuring patient safety.

Key Points

- Physicians are generally reluctant to assume the patient role. Barriers to care involve psychological resistance on the part of the physician, systemic factors stemming from stigmatization of psychiatric illness, and countertransference difficulties that mental health professionals have in treating physicians.

- Being diagnosed with a psychiatric disorder is not the same thing as being an "impaired physician."

- A clinician evaluating a physician must serve the patient and the safety of the public at the same time. Because of this complexity, the evaluator must strive to form an "evaluation alliance" with the patient.

- To assure the validity of the evaluation, as much collateral information as possible should be gathered from sources in the physician's family and in the workplace. Previous treatment records should also be obtained prior to the evaluation.

- The here-and-now behavior of the physician-patient during the evaluation often represents a repetition of the behavior at work that led to the evaluation.

PART II

Diagnostic and Treatment Issues in the Distressed and Distressing Physician

Psychiatric and Medical Illness in Physicians

In this chapter we discuss psychiatric and medical illnesses that are more commonly seen in physicians. As a group, physicians have been found to be healthier than the general population. Among both white and black men in the United States, physicians were older when they died and tended to die of the same causes as do others: heart and cerebrovascular disease and cancer (Frank et al. 2000). When death rates are compared, physicians are reported to have lower mortality rates for cancer and heart disease relative to the general population yet be at higher risk for suicide (Carpenter et al. 1997; Torre et al. 2000). Depression has been identified as a major risk factor for suicide (Holmes et al. 1990), and depression is reported to be as common in physicians as in the general population (Center et al. 2003). The same can be said about substance use disorders in physicians (Dilts and Gendel 2000).

Medical Illness in Physicians

In 1987, Mandell and Spiro wrote the following in the preface to their landmark book *When Doctors Get Sick*:

> Doctors get sick even as other people do. We doctors have no magical immunity
> to ward off devils or germs, whichever you think causes disease. People may not
> know that we ever get sick because we tend to work just the same unless the ill-
> ness is significantly debilitating. We physicians are in general a hardy lot and few
> of us stay home with the flu. This may not be good epidemiology but it helps to
> foster our superman and superwoman egos. (p. xi)

Although these words were written two decades ago, very little has changed in
the way that physicians face illness in themselves. Although doctors have been
publishing what it is like to be ill and to be a patient for years, Mandell and Spiro
were the first to co-edit a book on this subject. They compiled 50 first-person
accounts of physicians writing about their experience with cardiovascular diseases, orthopedic and neuromuscular disorders, neuropsychiatric disorders,
gastrointestinal diseases, cancer, chronic diseases, acute and self-limited diseases, and AIDS. All of the authors have much to say about the emotional sense
of being ill, the struggle with accepting the patient role, accessing medical care,
how they were cared for by their treating physicians, and the impact of their illnesses on their families and medical colleagues.

Doctors struggling with medical illness, especially illnesses that are disfig-
uring or otherwise visible, not uncommonly feel shunned by other physicians
(Rabin et al. 1982). Being shunned or perceiving shunning compounds stigma,
which adds to the burden of living with illness. Physicians, unlike the general
public, often feel stigmatized when they are living with illnesses not convention-
ally shameful, like diabetes, heart disease, cancer, and more. This seems to be
rooted in the sense of perfectionism and heartiness that characterizes the culture of medicine. To be ill is equated with weakness, being "less than," or, in the
idiom heard in some medical circles, not being able to "cut the mustard." This
is reinforced in medical settings that are not willing to accommodate a physician
who is now living with a partial disability and is no longer able to work a huge
number of hours per week, be as academically productive, or generate as much
income.

Psychiatrists who look after physicians who are living with an acute or
chronic medical illness can assist in many ways. The first and most pressing task
is to treat the emotional disorder that is accompanying or is a result of the medical disorder. The second is to reach out to the families of the physicians. Many
of them welcome the opportunity to discuss how the illness of their loved one is
affecting them and to pose questions that the psychiatrist, being medically
trained, may be able to answer. The third, and perhaps the most important, is
advocacy. Many physicians living with a medical disorder feel disappointed in, if
not enraged at, the insensitivity of their treating doctor (or team) to their personal and emotional needs. Compromised by illness and feeling too timid to
"rock the boat," many will be afraid to speak up to the treating physician(s). On
occasion, with the patient's permission, the treating psychiatrist may even con-

tact these physicians on their patient's behalf to explain the illness in more detail, review treatment options, discuss prognosis and the involvement of family members, and more. It is possible that the treating physician has not approached his or her physician-patient as a person first, physician second.

Chronic Medical Illness in Physicians

Case Example

Dr. Ward, a 43-year-old oncologist, was referred by her neurologist to a psychiatrist for assessment of fitness to practice. She had been diagnosed with multiple sclerosis (MS) during her residency 15 years earlier. Dr. Ward's disease had progressed significantly over the years, and her muscle weakness and neuropathic pain had necessitated her cutting back in her clinical duties. She had been working only 2 half-days per week in the local cancer clinic for the past 2 years, and now this workload even had become formidable.

"I'm very sad and pretty flat; I don't feel much anymore," said Dr. Ward in her opening statement. "I don't know if I'm clinically depressed or just grieving. My neurologist thinks that I'm giving in to my MS too much. He's always known me as a fighter. He thinks that I should take on more work, that I'm bored and have too much time on my hands to worry and what he calls 'indulge my disease.' I don't know what to think, I'm just confused."

The psychiatrist completed a very thorough psychiatric assessment. Although Dr. Ward had a depressed mood and other symptoms, she did not meet full criteria for a major depressive disorder. She was indeed grieving, as she had suggested. Psychotherapy was essential, and she improved markedly with the opportunity to talk about her many losses, fears for the future, and dreams and wishes of the things that she hoped to do in her foreshortened life. She was fit to practice, but she chose to retire and pursue some of her avocations.

This story touches on some of the themes that doctors living with a chronic illness face. The cutting short of a decades' long career after so many years of preparatory study and training can be hard. What is also a challenge is coming to terms with a career that may lack the luster that one had imagined. An example would be forfeiting what looked like a fast-track academic career while in residency, before being struck with the disease. Physicians can feel guilty when they feel angry or disappointed about "just being a simple clinician." These harsh inner feelings are magnified if colleagues make statements like "Just count your blessings; I have a patient who is already in a wheelchair, and he's only had MS for 7 years." Although remarks of this nature are patently insensitive, they are not unheard of in conversations with physician colleagues. Living with a chronic medical illness can be unbearably lonely and isolating in the world of medicine.

In addition to losses in one's professional life, there are personal defeats for physicians with chronic medical disease. There may be diminution of mobility that affects dexterity, freedom, and independence. Sports, travel, and play with children and grandchildren can suffer. Physicians who are single may find meeting eligible partners difficult. Sexuality may be a challenge and may lead to additional mourning. Most physicians know more about their prognosis or potential complications than lay people; thus, looking forward and visualizing even more assaults to their autonomy (which is especially precious in doctors) can be terrifying. Research on suicide in physicians identifies living with a chronic and progressively debilitating illness as a key risk factor (Center et al. 2003). It behooves the treating psychiatrist to explore notions of dying, euthanasia, and suicide with such patients. Most will welcome such frank discussions with a psychiatrist who is up to the journey.

Psychiatric Illness in Physicians

Case Example

"I'm broken," spoke Dr. Bates, a general internist, in his first visit to his psychiatrist. Intrigued and moved by his words and tone of voice, which was little more than a whisper, the psychiatrist asked him to explain further as he leaned forward to hear him. "It's physical and it's mental. I'm 46 years old by the calendar. My soul is 80. I look in the mirror and I see sagging defeat. My joints are wrong—they feel out of alignment, they're sore and painful and stiff—I've thought of a cane but that's too conspicuous because…I'm a shy man. The systems are slowed—circulatory, respiratory, digestive, and urinary—but thyroid function is normal. It's the brain and the mind that prompt this visit. Are they the same? I make a distinction. My brain is sluggish, it's not working right. Like I've had an infarct, a stroke without peripheral signs. Or that I'm hypoxic or have cerebral edema. Something is wrong, out of order. All I can do is guess. I've lost thoughts, words, sentences, gone—gone, I don't know where. The mind is worrying me. What mind? The mind is lost, devoid of spirit. It's like a flat tire, deflated, of no use any more. Can't be counted on. My brain thinks that my mind should be terrified about this. How I wish for that, for some emotion. But that's gone too, kaput. Maybe that's a big enough chief complaint. Forgive me for talking so much. Do you think you can help? I think I need more than glue."

This brief case vignette contains passages and inferences that are commonly embedded in the narratives of physician-patients:

- The word "broken" in his chief complaint speaks volumes. Dr. Bates uses it concretely, using phrases such as "sagging," "out of alignment," "like a flat tire," "in need of more than glue," but abstractly as well, using words like "defeat," "lost," "gone," and "no spirit." Different branches of medicine may use the word *broken* differently—for example, broken bones in orthopedic surgery, a broken heart valve or blood vessel in cardiology, broken skin in dermatology and plastic surgery—and it may be used in the questioning words of a psychiatrist-patient to her treating psychiatrist: "How broken is my brain?"

- The word "broken" can also have a mechanistic connotation that connects with the "fix it argument" that so many physicians use in defense of self-treatment: "I can fix this myself, I don't need to see a doctor." This is especially common in male physicians with troubled marriages. Their retort to their unhappy spouse who wants marital therapy is, "Can't we fix this ourselves? Why do we have to go see someone?" Rugged and self-reliant physicians look on their brokenness as a physical challenge akin to getting out their hammer or a set of wrenches.

- Dr. Bates uses medical jargon—words that convey meaning to his new psychiatrist, another physician, but words that are suggestive of intellectualization as a defense or what colloquially has been called "club language." Doctors use it at work and sometimes away from work. Club language can inadvertently distance physicians from each other.

- He uses the third person to describe some of his symptoms, as though he were presenting a patient to his psychiatrist: "The systems are slowed—circulatory, respiratory, digestive, and urinary...." Some physicians separate themselves from painful ownership of their brokenness by doing this. If Dr. Bates were a layperson, he would probably have used the first-person singular: "My whole body is slowing down—my heart, my breathing; I'm constipated, and I don't think that I'm passing as much urine as usual."

- Dr. Bates is clearly ill. He has probably been living with prodromal or early symptoms of illness for a while. He has delayed seeking help.

- He mentions normal thyroid function. Did he order his own thyroid stimulating hormone screening?

- He makes no reference to a primary care physician. Many doctors do not have one. It sounds as though he is self-referred in his statement "It's the brain and the mind that prompt this visit."

- There is a sense that Dr. Bates has been doing a lot of self-diagnosing and trying to rule things in and out. This is not uncommon in physician-patients, irrespective of their specialty, given their training in basic medicine.

- Dr. Bates's statement "I've thought of a cane but that's too conspicuous" prompts inquiry. Is it just that he is a shy man, or does he feel ashamed and humiliated that he is broken, ill, not as fit as his colleagues? Doctors abhor illness in themselves and tend to self-flagellate. Some doctor associates judge medical colleagues whom they perceive as flawed, and some ill physicians project their own self-judgment on to their associates.

- Dr. Bates says, "Forgive me for talking so much." This is the apology of so many ill physicians who come for help. It points to their interior sense of unworthiness. They view psychiatrists as very busy people, and they agonize that they are taking up precious time, time that should be spent tending to the "truly" mentally ill, like men and women with chronic schizophrenia and their homeless kin.

- Dr. Bates's whole presentation is very telling and common in physicians. His isolation and loneliness are palpable. He has so many symptoms, symptoms that he has been bearing with grace, with dignity. He is devoted to serving his patients and not worrying about his own needs. He does not want to bother anyone. His heavy sense of self resonates with the incisive words of Susan Sontag (1978): "Illness is the night side of life, a more onerous citizenship. Everyone who is born holds dual citizenship, in the kingdom of the well and in the kingdom of the sick" (p. 3). Physicians especially struggle with the notion of dual citizenship.

- Dr. Bates's descriptive sense of self is rich and layered. Not all patients consulting psychiatrists can speak so eloquently. This should be honored. Kendler (2005) has written: "The clinical work of psychiatry constantly requires us to assess and interpret the first-person reports of our patients. Many of the target symptoms that we treat can only be evaluated by asking our patients about their subjective experiences" (p. 433). When physicians become our patients they often present us with the fundamental questions of what it means to be human.

Determining Impairment

In Chapter 3 we discussed the problem of determining impairment in the context of a formal evaluation. It may be equally challenging in the course of an ongoing psychiatric treatment. Because most physicians who are consulting psychiatrists are conscientious and do not want to be working if they are at risk of making a mistake, some will raise this matter themselves early in treatment. Here is an example:

Case Example

Dr. Hill, a general surgeon, began his first visit to the psychiatrist with these words: "Thanks for seeing me so quickly. Something happened in the operating room last week that frightened me. I suddenly froze and stopped the procedure. My mind went blank as if I had passed out without losing consciousness. I came to, meaning I quickly realized where I was and that I was in the middle of a case. So I resumed what I was doing, a lymph node dissection. This occurred when my assistant asked if I was okay. Her words brought me back from wherever I was. I continued the operation uneventfully. I think I was only 'gone' a few seconds, but nevertheless it was weird. I'm not sure if I should be operating right now—and I haven't since this occurred. The stress in my life is astronomical at the moment. I've been dealing with a horrendous lawsuit that's dragged on for

5 years, but the biggest issue is that a month ago my wife left. I'm not handling that very well. I need your opinion on my safety."

Patients like Dr. Hill are easier to assess because the psychiatrist can work with their subjective sense of caution and support a voluntary leave until they are feeling better. Dr. Hill may be a patient who is able to conduct his office practice but is not completely safe in the operating room at this time. More difficult situations are ones in which the treating psychiatrist is concerned about the physician-patient's competence but the patient is not. Variables that determine whether the physician is open to a voluntary leave are the strength of rapport and therapeutic alliance, the degree of symptomatology, and the amount of insight that the physician-patient has. Collateral information is very helpful in sorting out whether the physician is capable of practicing. If concerns have been raised by medical colleagues or if there have been formal complaints, then the physician will have to accept that he or she cannot practice.

Depending on the branch of medicine and the various dimensions of the work that the person performs in a typical week, the patient may be able to continue working in a more limited way. For example, highly intensive manual work and mentally demanding tasks may need to be curtailed for awhile, but teaching, research, or administration may be manageable. What follows are examples of two different types of mood disorder and the kinds of symptoms that should be teased out in an ongoing treatment when trying to determine impairment.

Major Depressive Disorder

Many physicians living with an untreated or partially treated major depressive disorder are working and practicing medicine competently and safely. The symptoms that are most worrisome in terms of impairment are

- *Altered judgment due to severe melancholia.* It is very hard for doctor-patients to present a positive outlook regarding their patient's diagnosis or prognosis when their own mood is very gloomy or grim. Furthermore, if their appearance reveals their inner melancholia, this may frighten or worry their patients.
- *Lethargy.* Lethargy results in slowness to complete tasks in a timely way and tardiness. The doctor gets behind, delaying and irritating others, and this may compound an already compromised sense of self.
- *Trouble concentrating.* The doctor has trouble actively listening and following normal decision trees in clinical practice. Some complain that they can no longer "multi-task," an essential part of busy medical work.
- *Faulty memory.* This kind of memory loss is usually short term. The doctor asks the patient a question, only to be told that she had asked the same ques-

tion just 2 minutes earlier. This is embarrassing and inhibiting. Important medical information is missed or lost.

- *Guilty ruminations.* When physicians are struggling with this symptom, it may spill into their work. They have trouble being assertive with their patients and avoid directly confronting difficult or demanding patients. They may inappropriately and ponderously blame themselves for their patients not getting better in a timely manner or having an adverse outcome that is no one's fault but simply part of the disease.
- *Suicidal thoughts and actions.* Suicidal ideas and behaviors may be paramount in ill physicians' minds and preclude their being able to attend to their patient's concerns. They also may contaminate the doctor–patient relationship. Some suicidal physicians actually cross a boundary and disclose to their patient that they are feeling self-destructive. Their patients feel very frightened, responsible, or abandoned by their doctor about whom they now have to worry.

Hypomania or Mania

Few manic physicians are practicing medicine, and if they are, they should not be. Hypomania is another story, given that the field of medicine seems to applaud physicians with tremendous energy who work an enormous number of hours, treat lots of patients, fly off to medical meetings to present papers, attend functions with their spouses, and still play a mean game of tennis. The symptoms that are most worrisome in terms of impairment are

- *Expansive judgment due to euphoria or excitation.* Physicians with this symptom take on too much and do not tend to complete most of what they set out to do. It may be reinforced by colleagues who seem to need or feed off another physician's sunny disposition and creative energy. Hypomanic physicians may alienate others when they do not make meetings or deadlines because of overly committed schedules.
- *Heightened libido, possibly leading to sexual boundary violations.* This situation is very serious and constitutes a medical emergency. The physician should be put on medical leave before he or she destroys the doctor–patient relationship and his or her career with sexual misconduct.
- *Grandiose delusions that may also lead to boundary violations.* When physicians develop lofty ideas about their medical discoveries and treatment protocols or their great beauty and sexual desirability, they are prone to seductive behavior and ill-advised treatment with their patients.
- *Distraction and flightiness leading to tardiness, inappropriate actions, and errors.* These physicians are so wound up and easily distracted that they are late for surgery, office work, or lecturing trainees. The quality of their work suffers be-

cause they do not prepare properly or attend to the task at hand. They may make mistakes that range from minor to frankly dangerous.

- *Irritability that alienates colleagues and patients.* Touchiness and angry outbursts in the workplace upset and confuse others. This becomes a vicious circle when someone in authority attempts to speak to them or confront them about their actions. They lash out in response, because they have no capacity to see how they are acting and project any and all problems onto others.
- *Unprofessional behavior that may lead to shame later.* It is only when they are well that these doctors can look back and see how unlike their normal selves they had become when they were ill. Even if they can do their work safely and with competence (which may be debatable), they should still be deemed impaired because of how their behavior has an impact on colleagues. They will become isolated and marginalized—and may be fired.

Mood Disorders in Physicians: Unique Issues

A prospective study of medical students graduating from Johns Hopkins University found an overall 12% prevalence of depression (Ford et al. 1998). Frank and Dingle (1999) reported that 19.5% of U.S. female physicians have a history of depression. There is much anecdotal evidence of an increasing incidence of mood disorders in physicians, but it is speculated that this is because more physicians are seeking help than in the past, rather than a reflection of more new cases. We have no data on mood disorders in minority physicians or International Medical Graduates. Older resident data (Hendrie et al. 1990; Hsu and Marshall 1987) indicate that one-quarter to one-third of residents develop clinical symptoms of depression during their training. More recent data have found depression in up to 25% of medical students (Givens and Tija 2002).

Mood disorders in physicians cover the breadth of DSM-IV-TR (American Psychiatric Association 2000b), including major depressive disorder, bipolar I and II disorders, dysthymic disorder, mood disorder due to a medical condition, substance-induced mood disorder, and mood disorders that are comorbid with anxiety disorders, eating disorders, and so forth. There are many modes of presentation: the physician recognizes that she is ill and calls; the physician recognizes the symptoms but for various reasons cannot place the telephone call, so someone calls on his behalf; the physician begins to treat herself with antidepressant medication from office samples or self-prescribes; the physician consults his primary care physician for a seemingly medical condition with a range of somatic symptoms; the physician does not recognize or accept that she is ill and someone calls the psychiatrist for advice as to next steps; or the physician presents with overuse, abuse, or dependence on alcohol and/or other substances, and the diagnosis of a mood disorder is only uncovered after detoxification and initial recovery. Cocaine abuse may coexist with bipolar II disorder and may confuse the diagnostic picture.

Mood disorders in physicians may become manifest in still other ways. Some physicians report severe marital difficulty. They begin couples treatment, and the astute therapist uncovers an unrecognized and untreated mood disorder that is in part responsible for some of the marital discord. Or the therapist diagnoses depression in the physician that is secondary to unrelenting marital conflict and dysfunction. Some physicians develop suicidal ideation and begin to develop a plan for self-destruction. They do not always associate this type of thinking with depression. In some physicians, it is virtually ego-syntonic to think about suicide as a way out of suffering. All of this may lead to a suicide attempt, and the individual is brought to an emergency department. Suicide attempts in physicians tend to be very serious. Only a minority of doctors who die by suicide have made previous suicide attempts, as noted later in Chapter 11.

Finally, there are a number of physicians living with depression who present with behavioral change. Some examples include disruptive behavior in the medical workplace, especially when this change is de novo and truly out of character for the particular physician; sexual and nonsexual transgression of boundaries with patients; compulsive "cruising" in gay and bisexual male physicians that has become urgent and preoccupying and that puts them at great risk for professional ruin, sexually transmitted diseases, and violence; nonchemical "addictions" such as spending inordinate amounts of time on the Internet visiting porn sites, gambling, or engaging in compulsive spending and shopping; developing a "mid-life crisis" and suddenly leaving a spouse of 25 years for a partner who seems inappropriate in age or station in life; or any other risk-taking behaviors that point to a change or problem in judgment. Physicians coming to the attention of psychiatrists with any of these behavioral changes warrant a very thorough examination, including a careful assessment of mood.

Case Example[1]

Dr. Cowan and his wife presented for marital therapy. He was an infectious disease specialist and academic. His wife was a homemaker and community volunteer. They had three teenage sons. The initial visit with the psychiatrist began with a bang. Detained at the hospital with a suicidal patient, the psychiatrist was 5 minutes late. He apologized. Dr. Cowan looked at his watch and asked, "Will you be making up the time today or at the next visit, if there is one?" The psychiatrist apologized again and invited them to talk about their concerns. Mrs.

---

[1]This case, in part revised, was previously published in Myers 2002 and was adapted with permission of *Physician's Money Digest.*

Cowan seemed embarrassed and nervous; her speech was faltering and digressive. Dr. Cowan cut in with "Let me explain. We're here because my wife and her female psychiatrist think that I'm a 'control freak.' I don't totally disagree but I don't totally agree either. I am a very organized and exacting person—I don't suffer fools gladly. I didn't get to be a division chief at the age of 35 for no good reason. Meredith is different than me, aren't you dear? Quite laid back. Why do you bristle when I ask you about your day? Aren't you responsible for the running of the home? I just want to make sure that you're doing it properly."

The psychiatrist asked Mrs. Cowan to respond. She said "Here's how you ask about my day Peter—you don't even say hello or hug me like you used to. You walk in the back door and start with your laundry list: 'Did you water the flowers on the front deck? Why isn't the car in the garage? I thought you were going to call someone to get that gutter fixed? Why isn't Marcus practicing his violin? Who left the light on in the basement? You didn't bake another apple pie, did you—you know that Josh can't have any, he's really getting fat—what an enabler you are! I hope that you didn't forget the dry cleaning."

Not surprisingly, Dr. Cowan reacted defensively and with long explanations for all of his questions. He could not see that it was his manner that rankled. The psychiatrist got both of them off this subject in order to learn more about the history of their marriage and their kids. They brightened up, lightened up, and found some affection for each other. The visit ended on a better note than it began.

Their individual sessions with the psychiatrist were illuminating. Mrs. Cowan told the psychiatrist that her husband hated to go to bed alone. When she wanted to stay up later and held her ground, her husband got very upset, more demanding, and sometimes left the house angrily. This frightened her. When the psychiatrist met with Dr. Cowan, he took a detailed developmental history. Dr. Cowan was an only child and was revered by his somewhat older parents. He had childhood anxiety—his books and toys had to be "just so" before he got into bed; he slept with his nightlight on until university (and beyond); he fretted that his parents might divorce; he worried that he would fail an examination and not be number one in his class; he had very few friends; and he hated sports. "I was kind of a nerd, but what the hell, look what a success I've become." However, Dr. Cowan also had had an 8-week period of depression in medical school that was not treated. He improved spontaneously, but some symptoms returned about 1 year ago—intense irritability, a 10-pound weight loss that he passed off as deliberate, trouble falling off to sleep and early morning awakening, memory slippage, and crying spells that he was ashamed of and disclosed to no one.

The psychiatrist diagnosed atypical depression and prescribed antidepressant medication. Within 3 weeks, Dr. Cowan was calmer and less negative. He reported that he was sleeping better, including being able to sleep alone. He felt much less tense. Mrs. Cowan felt that she had her husband back. Marital therapy assisted with their communication pattern and intimacy struggles.

Dementia in Physicians

Dementia in a practicing physician is extraordinarily worrisome. Classically, these physicians have minimal to no insight into their cognitive decline, memory difficulties, disinhibition, and other deficits. In some medical settings, such as a solo private practice, a physician's illness may be covered up by a nurse or secretary who compensates by doing tasks normally done by the physician, making excuses, and checking for and correcting mistakes on orders, prescriptions, and accounting.

Case Example

A 79-year-old family physician, Dr. White, was referred to a psychiatrist because of "unusual actions" with his patients. The referring internist wondered if Dr. White should be practicing and hoped that he could be persuaded to retire. The complaints were informal and came to his internist by patients they had in common who were worried about Dr. White's health. He feared that if something were not done soon, Dr. White would harm a patient and be sued or that a patient might complain to the medical licensing board. The "unusual actions" included calling patients by the wrong name; forgetting what patients came to see him about; asking the same questions again and again; listening to the patient's chest (and talking the whole time) and not examining the abdomen when the complaint was lower abdominal pain; repeatedly telling his patients how despondent he felt since his wife's death 5 years earlier; appearing at work unshaven and in the same wrinkled clothes; and being slow and distracted, forcing his patients to wait up to 2 hours to see him.

The psychiatrist found Dr. White cooperative with the interview but unsure about why he was there. "I hear that people are worried about me, but I'm well, very well. I love my practice and my patients." When the psychiatrist told Dr. White what some of the concerns were, he was surprised, glib, and overly familiar: "Well, that's not so bad, I was really worried…it's good to know I haven't killed anyone—yet. Just kidding, Doc." On mental status examination, Dr. White was superficial, rambling, and perseverative in speech. He was emotionally labile, laughing at questions that were not particularly funny and becoming easily irritated with the psychiatrist's gentle probing and attempts to understand. He kept referring back to Clara, his wife, and how much he missed her. He cried a lot. He was not oriented to date or day of the week. He could not get past 93 on serial sevens. He knew the name of the president but gave the names of past presidents in order as Ford, Clinton, and Eisenhower. He refused tests of similarities with an angry defensive statement: "Now you're trying to insult me…I'm not going to let you…I'm older and a lot smarter than you."

The psychiatrist summed up at the end and told Dr. White that he was worried about him and wanted him to take a voluntary medical leave from his practice. He told Dr. White that he thought he was depressed on top of a painful grief reaction and that he needed treatment for that. He also pointed out his cognitive and memory difficulties and suggested that they needed detailed investigation by a neurologist. He said, "Although you can get impaired thinking and memory with depression, which we will treat, I want to make sure there isn't something organic going on. This is why I don't want you to work right now. You have had a long and very successful career and it would be terrible if you made a serious medical error and harmed someone. Wouldn't you agree?" Dr. White agreed and only mildly protested, "But I can't go on sick leave. Who will look after my patients?" The psychiatrist volunteered to contact the local physician health program, and a locum physician was found.

Dr. White never returned to work. He accepted the neurologist's diagnosis of early dementia with equanimity. His son and daughter, both very supportive and relieved, were very helpful with this transition and organized his personal healthcare needs.

Psychosis in Physicians

Doctors are vulnerable to psychotic illness as much as anyone else. There is perhaps one exception to this axiom—schizophrenia. Because of its usual early onset, a young person wanting to pursue medicine would probably have had a first episode in college and would have to rethink applying to medical school. If already in medical school, students with schizophrenia would have difficulty completing their studies because of the serious nature of their illness. Nevertheless, cases of schizophreniform illnesses are not unheard of in physicians. Probably the most common psychoses in physicians are ones that accompany mood disorders, substance use disorders, and medical illness. Delusional disorder is also far from rare.

Case Example

Dr. Singh was a third-year resident in pathology who was referred for assessment by his training director after he assaulted another resident in his office at one of the local teaching hospitals. Dr. Singh had confronted Dr. Jones with accusations that the latter was stealing data from Dr. Singh's research project on pediatric leukemia. Dr. Jones was aghast and denied all of the charges against him, which made Dr. Singh even more angry and threatening. Dr. Jones asked him to leave but he refused. A scuffle ensued, and Dr. Singh slugged Dr. Jones and knocked him to the ground. Others heard this and called security. Dr. Singh was detained and told to go home and relax. He met with the training director the next day and was put on leave pending an evaluation.

The initial visit began thus: "I have come to see you because I need your help. It's my program director who is insisting that you look me over. I don't need a psychiatric assessment, but I do need your help. I pray that you can get to the bottom of this departmental conspiracy against me. I know that sounds very paranoid, but it is not paranoia. I am not the problem—they are. I have felt uncomfortable in this residency since day one when I reported to work. See my turban? I'm Sikh. They do not like Indians in this program. I have proof that I am not being advanced like the 'white' residents. Let me show you what I have here in my attaché case. See these six report books? I have a complete log of the comings and goings in this department from that day forward. No one knows of this."

The psychiatrist asked him to explain the altercation with Dr. Jones: "It's very simple. He's a liar and a very clever one at that. His research is also in pediatric blood dyscrasias but not leukemia. His area is sickle cell disease. But I have templates on my computer that he has modified to fit his project. He's a psychopath. I don't need to tell you how smart and manipulative psychopaths are. He somehow got my password several weeks ago. When I saw that my data were transgressed, I knew immediately it was him. I didn't confront him though. I just very casually and with innocent surprise mentioned to him that someone had been surfing my research files. I watched his face out of the corner of my eye. He smiled ever so slightly and said with false sincerity 'You're kidding.' He acted concerned, but I'm wise to his BS. Anyway, despite changing my password twice since, he gained access. And that is why I decided to let him have it. I'm tired of being a victim. And I'm pretty sure he is not acting alone. I have some suggestive evidence but not foolproof facts—yet."

Thorough assessment of Dr. Singh over a series of interviews, with collaborative information (with his permission) from his training director and from his very worried family, concluded that he had a delusional disorder. He refused treatment when neuroleptic medication was suggested. When several months passed without the patient returning for care, Dr. Singh was dismissed from his residency. Although he threatened a wrongful dismissal complaint, he did not pursue this. At last report, he was living at home with his parents and working for his brother-in-law in his construction business.

Anxiety Disorders in Physicians

A significant number of physicians with mood and substance use disorders have a concurrent anxiety disorder that is not always evident at first. Only with some improvement in the patients' mood do the anxiety symptoms become more obvious. Similarly, scores of physicians in early recovery from alcohol and opioid (and other drug) abuse are found to have an underlying anxiety disorder that they either did not know they had, or if they once did know, they had been self-medicating with drugs for so long that they had forgotten.

However, doctors can have stand-alone anxiety disorders on Axis I. Generalized anxiety disorder can be embarrassing for trainees and physicians who have visible tremors, widened pupils, sweating, cold hands, diarrhea, urinary frequency, and more during rounds, in clinical teaching units, and in their offices. Physicians with social anxiety disorder may come for help when it becomes evident that they are avoiding preparing grand rounds or presenting cases at the bedside; their shyness and social inhibition may be making dating impossible. Physicians with posttraumatic stress disorder may present after being sexually harassed at work, assaulted by a patient, or the victim of a home invasion. Physicians with obsessive-compulsive disorder (OCD) may come for help if their symptoms become crippling and impair their work performance.

Case Example

Dr. Kelly, a first-year resident in psychiatry, gave the following chief complaint to her psychiatrist: "Thank you for seeing me. I think that I have OCD. Well I know I have OCD, I've had it all my life. But it's become a problem. I'm spending more and more time with my rituals, and I'm going to get in trouble for being late for work in the morning. One of my supervisors has already picked up on it. The truth is that I can't get out of the house in the morning in less than 2 hours. I've been setting my alarm earlier and earlier, which means I'm getting less sleep because I'm a bit of a night owl." Dr. Kelly's thoughts and compulsive behaviors were a mix of counting and checking. In the morning, after a timed shower and very idiosyncratic shampooing and rinsing ritual, she had to repeat the entire procedure. Dressing was straightforward if she laid out her clothes the night before, but fixing her hair took time. She had to arrange her papers and books once each morning and quickly vacuum her rug. Only once. Then she had to sit and listen carefully to a specific Bach fugue 3 mornings a week. "But," she said cheerfully, "At least I don't have to check the burners and the door and car locks like my patient. …I know this may seem weird to you, but because I am spared those rituals, I don't feel quite so screwed up."

Dr. Kelly did very well with treatment. This included a moderate dosage of a selective serotonin reuptake inhibitor medication prescribed and monitored by her psychiatrist and cognitive-behavioral therapy conducted by a psychologist. Over the course of several months she was able to let go of a number of her repetitive behaviors and greatly reduce the number of bathing and grooming steps in the morning. This gave her great relief, and her self-esteem improved. She was consistently on time—or early— for work, and her outstanding in-training evaluations reinforced the importance of self-care and adherence to treatment.

Biopsychosocial Treatment Principles

In Chapter 3 we advised that evaluations must take into account both biological and psychosocial factors. The same comprehensiveness must apply to treatment planning and implementation.

Biological Factors

Because many doctors do not have primary care physicians and refer themselves directly to psychiatrists, it is important to consider biological factors in their illness. Taking a detailed family history will uncover genetic predisposition to many psychiatric illnesses, especially mood disorders and substance dependence, both of which can increase the risk of suicide. A review of systems will facilitate a consideration of medical factors—metabolic, endocrine, infection, malignancies, cardiovascular, and more—that may be contributing to symptom genesis. Concerns about dementia will be dictated by age (Alzheimer's), habits (HIV, smoking), and other causes (head trauma). Asking about prescribed drugs and self-medicating is important (e.g., propranolol, benzodiazepines, antihypertensives, Accutane) both at the outset of treatment and during its course. Most important, a detailed inquiry about alcohol and street drug (e.g., cocaine, cannabis, ketamine) abuse is essential.

Medical factors must be addressed. If the doctor-patient does not have a general physician, the psychiatrist or therapist may need to encourage, if not insist upon, a workup for physical causes of the presenting problems. Also, some patients do not have a treating physician who is at arm's length and who can provide objective care; they have chosen their medical partner or even a family member who is a doctor. Probing often reveals that there is no official medical record (because they work in the same office) and no full history or physical examination has ever been completed. This problem should be discussed, and consent should be obtained to enable the psychiatrist to communicate with other caregivers about important medical investigations, concomitant medical disorders, and other medications that the physician-patient is taking. A word of caution: most physician-patients are comforted by the treating psychiatrist who is very judicious in what he or she discloses (in both oral and written form) to other caretakers about the reason for psychiatric treatment. The diagnosis and drug treatment are acceptable, but psychodynamic details and current conflicts may be omitted. This gives the physician-patient some measure of privacy and helps to safeguard trust and confidentiality in the medical world in which he or she works.

Depending on the diagnosis, a range of somatic treatments may be necessary: antidepressants (monotherapy, augmentation strategies, combination treatment), second-generation neuroleptics, mood stabilizers, appropriate medications for anxiety and/or sleep disturbance, and occasionally electroconvulsive therapy for severe depression. Individuals with concurrent substance dependence will need treatment by an addiction physician. The pharmacological treatment of mood disorders can be difficult, and state-of-the-art drug treatment is essential. Treating psychiatrists may have to accept the limits of their knowledge and obtain a second opinion. Any physician with a treatment-resistant mood disorder should be referred to a skilled psychopharmacologist for a consultation, even if this involves seeing someone at a distance. This decision is dictated by the enhanced morbidity (i.e., suffering, family strain, inability to work) and mortality (risk of suicide) of severe mood disorders in physicians. Some psychiatrists develop negative countertransferences and start blaming their physician-patients for not trying hard enough to get better when the patients have clearly been undertreated.

Self-medicating needs to be discussed, and all prescribing should be done by the treating physician. Using office samples of medication is strongly discouraged by many psychiatrists. Others will accept it, provided that the physician-patient is only taking medications that are prescribed by the psychiatrist, not medications that are similar or of the same class. This tendency to trade one medication for another is common in doctors and must be discussed. Other matters that warrant discussion include stopping medications when the patient thinks they can be stopped, not renewing medications, self-prescribing because "I didn't want to bother you," increasing and decreasing dosages without telling the treating physician, and so forth. Physicians are competitive by nature, and often those who are dutiful and compliant in person will enact competitive transference issues *outside* the sessions by adjusting medications on their own. Respecting how side effects influence treatment adherence is key, as is psychoeducation. We have found that psychoeducation is especially important when the patient is a psychiatrist, but this must be done with care and respect. Too often the psychiatrist neglects this aspect of care altogether, assuming that the physician-patient already knows the side effects of the medication!

Psychological Factors

Loss

Loss, both recent and past, is not uncommon in physicians who present for psychiatric treatment. Sometimes it is a causative factor and contributes to the illness: loss of a loved one by death, separation, or divorce; loss of well-being and physical stamina in previously well and fit physicians; loss of status and stature in an academic setting; and loss of sameness and certainty when physicians move geographically or divorce. Many physicians live their lives with aggregate loss; they are walking around with much unrecognized and unresolved grief for the loss of a parent in medical school, a loss of a patient, of former spouse(s), of other loved ones and friends, of pets, of youth, or of sexual confidence and function.

The "busyness" of medicine precludes, distorts, or mocks normal grieving. Sometimes loss is a result of the illness itself—loss of happiness, strength, efficiency, task completion, and life chances; loss of intimacy—emotional, intellectual, sexual; loss of self-esteem and resilience; loss of confidence in one's judgment; loss of hope and predictability; loss of the ability to practice medicine or work at level of one's training and job experience; loss of professional connections; loss of career trajectory; loss of finances from limited ability to work, medical leave, bad investments, and reckless spending if hypomanic or manic; and finally, loss of respect due to stigma. This pervasive sense of loss may become apparent only after the patient is in treatment and "sits still" long enough to reflect.

Trauma

An unknown number of physicians are at risk for psychiatric illness because of childhood trauma. They may be victims of abuse (e.g., physical, sexual, or emotional), and this contributes to the adult illnesses of posttraumatic stress disorder, eating disorders, and mood disorders. Psychiatrists and physicians who do a lot of psychological counseling and therapy in their practices may present with *vicarious traumatization* (McCann and Pearlman 1990). This term refers to how a therapist reacts to and processes painful and graphic material that traumatized patients bring to treatment. Residents have described trauma during training in the form of aggressive and shaming teachers, verbal or sexual harassment, treating victims of family violence, and coping with horrific trauma in emergency department settings. Acute stress disorder may progress to post-traumatic stress disorder in vulnerable physicians and if brief crisis intervention has not been offered or prescribed in the medical setting. Like the effects of loss, the impact of trauma may not be apparent until well into the treatment.

Case Example

Dr. Pilsner grew up in the rural South, where the saying "Spare the rod, spoil the child" was oft repeated. When he was 51, he sought out psychotherapy for the first time in his life because of depression and anxiety. When asked if he had a history of abuse, he responded, "No, nothing like that. My father used to whip my ass with a belt until there were welts, but that was the same as what the other kids got." This minimization of the traumatic whippings finally dissolved when he sobbed uncontrollably in a session while discussing his deep sense of self-loathing. In the midst of his tears, he said, "My father beat it into me that I was a worthless piece of shit." This episode emerged 6 months into the therapy after layers of defense gave way to the realization that the whippings had destroyed his self-esteem.

Ongoing and Unrelenting Stress and Conflict

Examples of ongoing stress include the everyday concerns of medical practice, marriage, and worries about children. These are dimensions of the physician's life that may cause him or her to break out into symptoms.

Any type of psychotherapy may be indicated for these patients: supportive, interpersonal, cognitive-behavioral, psychodynamic, and more. Modalities include individual, couple, family, and group. Social therapies range from Alcoholics Anonymous groups to various experiential and humanistic types of help. Most treating psychiatrists are not versed in a large range of therapies, and many doctor-patients will need referrals to other professionals for this kind of assistance. Details of these therapies are discussed later in this volume. Many physicians can benefit from a range of personal and work hygiene suggestions by their psychiatrist: encouraging lifestyle changes as necessary, reducing the number of hours worked each week, exercising, ensuring adequate rest each day, booking reasonable vacation time each year, eating healthy foods, drinking less alcohol, and supporting spiritual and religious exploration.

Social and Cultural Factors

There are many issues that are contemporaneous in doctors' lives that may contribute to their symptoms. Some of these may be remote but nonetheless toxic and warrant examination and psychological exploration.

- *Workplace and community strain (e.g., persistent stress without a solution, entrapment, unrelenting harassment).* Residents and fellows, for example, may have no other option but to remain in the specific setting of training. They survive by knowing that there is an endpoint. International Medical Graduates and many minority physicians may also believe that they have no other option but to remain where they are.
- *Financial worries in chronically ill doctors who can only work part-time.* There are many work settings that have not accepted the notion of residual disability. They want physicians who are 100% well and functioning. Many of these doctors struggle to accept their limitations in an unforgiving work culture.
- *Racism, bigotry, sexism.* Like it or not, many physicians are victims of discrimination. In academic settings, there may be a human resources department available. In many settings there may be no place to turn. Treating psychiatrists need to listen attentively to their patient's narratives of discrimination.
- *Religious persecution.* Some physicians in North America have fled forces that are hostile to their faith. Their host country may be more embracing, but it may take time to build trust.
- *Social homophobia and gay bashing.* Not all gay and lesbian physicians feel comforted by a more accepting stance in the house of medicine. Some are victims of abuse outside of the medical workplace. This strain can contribute to a multitude of forces that make a physician feel ill or behave inappropriately at work.

Advocacy Strategies

Being an advocate for one's patient is fundamental in psychiatry, but it is especially important when treating physicians. There are many situations in which the psychiatrist can advance the patient's restoration of health by inquiry and speaking out, including interviewing family members, friends, and medical co-workers (with the patient's consent); listening to the concerns of associate deans, program directors, department heads, medical directors, licensing board officials, disability insurance physicians, rehabilitation consultants, primary care physicians, other medical specialists, and any other mental health professionals who have been involved; communicating with the state/provincial physician health program; conveying key information/updates to select personnel (again with appropriate permission); and accompanying the patient to meetings with his or her training director or chief of staff.

All of these advocacy positions must be cautiously considered if the treating clinician is conducting psychotherapy with the physician. The frame of the therapy can be seriously compromised if the patient knows that what is discussed in therapy may be repeated to a third party. Under such circumstances some physician-patients may conceal aspects of their situation that will place them in unfavorable light. Moreover, an advocate role may make it difficult for the psychotherapist to confront the patient about abrasive interpersonal behavior, dishonesty, narcissism, and other behaviors. Sometimes being a good therapist entails explaining to physician-patients why they are *not* ready to resume full responsibilities.

Education of others is a central part of treating physicians with both medical and psychiatric disorders. This approach serves to correct outdated views about various illnesses in physicians and works to diminish stigma in medicine. Education informs others that some of the most talented and gifted physicians in North America live with a well-treated psychiatric disorder (Myers and Dickstein 1999–2007). Education also informs others that psychiatric disorders are serious and that some doctors, with the best of care, will have to live with residual symptoms and can only work part-time.

Other advocacy work includes offering and giving telephone consultations to people in authority who are concerned about a physician in their midst and do not know what to do; making oneself available to assess quickly physicians who are highly symptomatic; volunteering to give "psychiatric updates" (e.g., grand rounds) to one's nonpsychiatrist medical colleagues; watching for instances of physician abuse in medical settings and speaking out or writing letters of concern; and supporting physicians who are interested yet hesitant to write about their own personal struggle with mental illness.

The following is the first-person account of a middle-aged psychiatrist who has had three episodes of major depressive disorder in the past and who was in remission at the time of this writing.

> Churchill called it the "Black Dog." For me it is the black ball—a dense, heavy cannon ball about the size of a fist that sits in the pit of my stomach. Often it appears first, before the empty, aching sense of dread that inevitably follows. I fantasize that if I were to be operated on, the surgeon could remove this tumor and I would feel light and free. It feels like a physical illness, and even a hot water bottle makes it feel better. Soon, though, energy drops away and I lie curled up like an invalid.
>
> What follows, surprisingly, is crystal-clear insight. It is completely obvious that my entire life has been a complete failure and that I have screwed up every aspect of it. There is no hope for the future, and things will only get worse. Life is utterly pointless, and there is no pleasure in anything nor any hope of change. Happiness is an illusion. Despair is real. The next phase is the fantasy of ending things for good, and planning begins, quite comforting really, like playing with worry beads. Ask for help? Why would I? There is no hope, everything is completely pointless, and they would just try to change my mind when I know my analysis of the situation is absolutely correct. I wouldn't want to worry friends or family, and I would hate to be a bother.
>
> Then, like a fever, the acute phase breaks, and I mope around in a blue funk grumbling and moaning inside about how useless and stupid life is. The anger

gets directed at the world and the maybe God who created it and now I feel like the victim, not the cause. A couple of weeks later and things are back to normal, and sometimes I even think how fortunate I am…until the next time.

Key Points

- Physicians are human and subject to the same range of medical and psychiatric illnesses as the general public. Because of knowledge and some adherence to a healthy lifestyle, they are less likely to have some illnesses but have high rates of substance abuse and dependence, mood disorders, and suicide.

- Because stigma, overwork, and denial of one's vulnerability loom large in the house of medicine, many physicians do not take good care of themselves or seek timely medical attention when they are ailing.

- Although the road to treatment may be delayed and circuitous, once physicians become patients and accept their need for care, they often are exemplary patients. This offsets the cynicism shown toward physicians that they act entitled and are difficult and demanding patients.

- Applying the time-honored biopsychosocial approach when assessing and treating physicians will yield the best results and greatly enhance prevention.

- The treating psychiatrist can assist many physician-patients by advocating on their behalf. Physicians who are ill—and those on the mend—can be very intimidated by medical authority figures, and the expertise and experience of their treating psychiatrist will greatly facilitate their return to work. This action not only reassures the doctor-patient but also educates employers and others in power, resulting in greater understanding and compassion.

Addictions

Chemical and Nonchemical

The following are statements culled from the practices of psychiatrists specializing in the field of physician health:

> "We've come to see you for three reasons—we're fighting a lot, we're each working too damn hard, and we're both drinking too much." (Dr. Monroe and Dr. Gardner)
>
> "I guess my program director already spoke to you. Someone smelled alcohol on my breath last weekend when I was on call. Let me explain." (Dr. Winston, Senior Resident, Obstetrics and Gynecology)
>
> "This is Mrs. Wallace calling. Would you be willing to see my husband and me? My husband's a psychiatrist. I'm really worried about him—he's depressed, and I think he's becoming or already is an alcoholic. He told me he won't come to see you, but I think that I can get him to your office if we come together for our marriage."
>
> "Am I upset? How would you feel if you went home from work tonight and your wife and kids had moved out? All that's there is a note 'Don't even bother to contact us until you've dealt with your drinking problem.'" (Dr. Alton)
>
> "I'm just back from a treatment center. Three months. I've been diagnosed with polyaddictions—alcohol, gambling, and Internet pornography—and depression and a personality disorder. I'm seeing Dr. Suitor for my addictions but I need a psychiatrist too. I need to get my license back, and I want my wife back too." (Dr. Palmerston)

Research suggests that physicians are no more likely to have a substance use disorder (especially alcohol abuse and dependence) than socioeconomically matched professionals serving as control subjects (Mansky 2004). However, some data (Hughes et al. 1992) indicate that physicians may be more likely to abuse prescription drugs because of their greater accessibility. The lifetime incidence of a substance use disorder in physicians ranges from 8% to 15% (Coombs 1997), and alcohol is the most commonly abused drug. Prescribed drugs of abuse include opiates, benzodiazepines, other sedatives and hypnotics, and stimulants (amphetamines and methylphenidate). Recently, Gold et al. (2004, 2006) reported that anesthesiologists, surgeons, and emergency physicians are overrepresented among physician opiate addicts. Street drugs abused by doctors include cannabis, cocaine, ecstasy, and ketamine ("Special K"). When a physician is chemically dependent, use of more than one drug, or *polysubstance abuse,* is not uncommon. Variables that account for some of the differences in physician drug abuse include the presence of concurrent medical and psychiatric illness, one's branch of medicine and easy availability of certain medications, gender, age, geographical location, race, and ethnicity.

Case Example

Dr. Sprott was a 36-year-old internist who was referred for psychiatric consultation by a neurologist. She had been admitted to the neurology unit 48 hours earlier, having been brought to the hospital by ambulance after having had a grand mal convulsion at home. She was disoriented and agitated, with both auditory and visual illusions. Investigation for a seizure disorder revealed that Dr. Sprott had been self-medicating with up to 16 mg of lorazepam daily. Because of insomnia, she was also drinking up to 8 oz. of vodka through the night. To counteract the tiredness and fatigue during the day, she started to take "diet" pills several months earlier. Fully cognizant of the risk of a withdrawal syndrome, she nonetheless had decided to go "cold turkey" and stop all her medications (except her self-prescribed tricyclic antidepressant) a couple of days prior to admission.

Once her delirium cleared and she began receiving a slowly tapered dosage of benzodiazepines, her psychiatrist learned that she had first seen a psychiatrist in college for severe anxiety and pan-phobias. In medical school, she had her first depressive illness but did not seek help. "I was scared that the dean would find out and this would affect my getting into a good residency. I toughed it out." Once she got her medical license and entered residency she began to write prescriptions for herself. "As I got more and more into my addiction, I got deeper and deeper into my shame." Dr. Sprott acknowledged to her psychiatrist that she felt relieved to be in treatment.

Unfortunately, this case is not atypical and is illustrative of how physicians with addictions often use poor judgment and take extreme risks with their health. Dr. Sprott had no untoward complications of her delirium nor her withdrawal seizure. Although she acknowledged the presence of anxiety symptoms as far back as her undergraduate days, she balked at seeking proper psychiatric care during medical school and beyond. Given the availability of medical services on many medical campuses and their commitment to confidential care, some might find her sense of stigma overdetermined. Nevertheless, many contemporary trainees who develop psychiatric symptoms will not come forward for help, putting themselves at risk of feeling worse and self-prescribing.

Biopsychosocial Determinants of Addiction

Genetic predisposition has long been known to be a risk factor for individuals developing alcoholism and other types of substance abuse. Twin studies have provided the strongest evidence that experiential conditions play an important role and that environmental conditions and processes influence the risk of developing dependence on alcohol and other drugs (Anthony and Chen 2004). Estimates of heritability for alcohol dependence and other drug dependence range from 25% to 65%. This leaves considerable room for the influence of noninherited characteristics in the genesis of addiction. In most studies, the estimated contribution of nongenetic familial transmission tends to be notably smaller than the estimated contribution of individual-specific (nonshared) environmental causes. The genes that influence initiation of use have a very strong effect on the ultimate risk of abuse, and they are largely nonspecific for the class of drug (Cloninger 2004). Exploration of the genetics of substance abuse is a dynamic and ever-evolving endeavor that will ultimately help to explain why some physicians are more at risk for substance dependence than others and what role personality plays in this process.

A significant number of physicians come from families in which one or more first-degree relatives have a substance abuse or dependence problem. Indeed, we know from family systems research on drug dependence that various immediate family members assume or are assigned roles, one of which is caretaker or rescuer. When a child or adolescent gains experience with this task, he or she may become interested in studying medicine. Others pursue medicine with a need for mastery, to research or even "cure" a disease that has hit very close to home.

Other biological underpinnings for developing a substance use disorder are medical illnesses that have made the physician quite symptomatic. Examples include rheumatoid arthritis, cancer, diabetes, multiple sclerosis, back pain and other types of pain syndromes, orthopedic injuries, chronic fatigue syndrome, and more. Unlike laypersons, who return to their treating physicians when they have unrelenting pain or anxiety or other forms of discomfort, many physicians begin to drink heavily for the first time, drink more, or self-prescribe medication. Some obtain higher and higher amounts of opiates and benzodiazepines from their treating physicians, who unwittingly enable the overuse of controlled substances in their doctor-patients. Iatrogenic substance dependence is not rare in physicians.

Some physicians living with psychiatric illness develop a chemical dependency from trying to treat their symptoms. Those at highest risk are physicians with a preexisting vulnerability to substance abuse and physicians whose psychiatric disorder is unrecognized, confusing, or mysterious. In other words, they do not realize that they have obsessive-compulsive disorder (OCD), posttraumatic stress disorder, or a social anxiety disorder. What they notice is that they feel better or more confident after a couple of drinks, after smoking cannabis, or after taking oxycodone or their spouse's sleeping medication. Even when physicians are in active treatment with a psychiatrist, they may not disclose their higher use of alcohol or use of psychotropic samples from the office to alleviate untreated symptoms. The psychiatrist may even foster substance use in the physician-patient if he or she concludes inappropriately that the patient's illness is treatment resistant and that the patient must accept a partial response to treatment; the physician-patient thus is left with little alternative but to treat him- or herself.

Exciting neurobiological research is under way in addictions. A common molecular pathway in the brain has been ascribed to addiction (Nestler 2005). Emerging concepts suggest that addictions converge on a common circuitry in the limbic system, the mesolimbic dopamine pathway (Tamminga and Nestler 2006). All drugs of abuse increase dopamine release in the nucleus accumbens, and many also stimulate the release of endogenous opioid peptides in this region. Drugs induce a long-term potentiation-like state in ventral tegmental area dopamine neurons and a long-term depression-like state in nucleus accumbens neurons. Broader brain circuits mediate addiction, including the amygdala, hippocampus, and frontal cortex, which are all parts of the brain's memory systems. Human addiction involves powerful emotional memories and is increasingly known to be a disorder of the brain's reward system.

These findings, coupled with functional imaging studies, aid in explaining relapse in physicians with substance dependence. In a study of 292 physicians reported by Domino et al. (2005), one in four monitored doctors relapsed at least once. The fact that well-trained and successful physicians do so—thus risking their licenses, livelihoods, and identities—provides circumstantial evidence that the drive to relapse originates far from conscious intent (Gastfriend 2005). Risk factors for relapse include genetic vulnerability, concurrent psychiatric disorder, specific psychosocial stressors, and type of substance. In physicians with major opioid use, dual diagnosis, and family predisposition (strong family history of substance use disorder), the risk of relapse was elevated 13-fold!

Mansky (1999) proposed a number of risk factors for physicians that may contribute to developing a substance use disorder. The following are based on clinical experience with addicted physicians and await empirical validation:

1. *Pharmacological optimism and knowledge.* Physicians witness how much medications help their patients quickly and often in life-saving situations. It may be tempting, especially in high-intensity branches of medicine, to seek the same kind of rapid response to personal angst by self-administering certain drugs.

2. *Reliance on intellectual abilities.* Being smart is essential for clinical decision making and practicing state-of-the-art medicine. However, in a paradoxical and self-defeating way, this use of intellect is considered to have a negative effect on the recognition of and recovery from a substance use disorder. Physician-patients may use their intellect to convince the naive or unsuspecting clinician that they are not dependent on alcohol and deny how their drinking is affecting their medical colleagues and family members. They may know how to get around random urine testing or give plausible reasons for missing appointments.

3. *Strong will.* Determination helps individuals to gain entrance to medical school and to cope with the rigors of everyday medical practice. However, this same trait in chemically dependent physicians can block recognition that a substance has taken hold and that one is indeed addicted. These physicians argue that they can stop and start alcohol or other drugs easily without tolerance or withdrawal and that they are nothing like the patients with end-stage addictions whom they look after.

4. *Love of challenges.* Some medical students and physicians have a history of taking risks and are sensation seekers. This may be rewarded in some programs that are extremely competitive and to which many people would not even bother applying. Furthermore, being seen as a "renaissance man or woman" by medical colleagues and superiors is reinforcing and can put an individual at risk for experimenting with drugs that can be dangerous or addicting.

5. *Instrumental use of drugs.* The classic story is the physician who uses amphetamines to cram for examinations in college and medical school. This may develop into using benzodiazepines during stressful times in residency or into using opiates to treat headaches, sports injuries, and other painful syndromes. Not uncommon is "deserving a big drink" after a long case in the operating room or a tough night on call.

6. *Denial.* So-called adaptive denial is healthy and essential in physicians. It enables the doctor to do his or her daily work with clinical neutrality, measured objectivity, and empathy so that patients benefit. Pathological denial occurs when physicians can no longer see that their use of alcohol or other substances is quantitatively or qualitatively abnormal and meets diagnostic criteria of a substance use disorder.

Other psychosocial determinants of addiction in physicians include the following:

1. *Overwork.* Working hard and for long hours has become normative in the house of medicine. When physicians return home at 7 P.M. or later, they may feel too tired to prepare a good meal or go to the gym. Winding down often includes one or more unmeasured drinks in front of the television or the newspaper. This can be reinforced by a spouse who also likes to drink. Physicians who are on their own may neglect their nutrition, at least during the week. These same doctors also argue that they are too busy to make an appointment to see their own primary care physician. It is easier to treat their symptoms in their own way.

2. *Entitlement.* "I've worked very hard today and I deserve a good drink" is the classic refrain.

3. *Ready access to medications.* Having pharmaceutical samples in one's office and the privilege of writing prescriptions are risk factors for addicted physicians.

4. *Cultural sanction.* Physicians who work in a milieu where most colleagues drink—or in the case of younger physicians, experiment with drugs—have enormous difficulty recognizing that their personal use of a drug has become excessive. Some even fear being ostracized should they decide on their own or at their doctor's suggestion to stop drinking.

5. *Stigma.* In its early stages, self-treatment with alcohol or other drugs is private, a secret. Physicians do not have to confront how ashamed they feel about consulting a colleague for anxiety or depression, an unhappy marriage, or a sexual orientation conflict. They can obtain some respite from their symptoms and preserve their autonomy at the same time by treating themselves. The tragic irony is that when the addicted physician does seek help, he or she is living with even more shame.

6. *Aging.* Studies of men and women postretirement have documented an increased use of daily or weekly alcohol use (Atkinson 1998; Brody 2002). Included in this group are physicians, especially doctors who are on their own, in loveless marriages, whose children (and perhaps grandchildren) live far away, and who are living with some of the common maladies of advancing age.

Case Example[1]

A psychiatrist received a telephone call from the 33-year-old son of Dr. and Mrs. Smythe. His words were, "My sister and I are really worried about our mom and

---

[1]This vignette is a revised version of a case previously published in Myers 2004. Adapted with permission of *Physician's Money Digest*.

dad. Since he's retired, the two of them have become a couple of drunks." At his request, the doctor met with him and his sister for more information. He learned that Dr. Smythe was age 68 and had retired from a career in radiology 3 years previously. Mrs. Smythe was the same age and a former nurse, mother, and homemaker. Her children described her as an alcoholic for many years, albeit in denial and never open to getting an assessment or being treated. They did not know when she had last seen a physician.

They described their father as codependent and an enabler of their mother's drinking. Over the years, he placated them when they tried to talk about her use of alcohol. His own father had died of cirrhosis, so he would drink only minimally—until recently. Now, his speech was often slurred when he called, and they found empty gin bottles in the trunk of his car and a stash of liquor hidden in the workshop on their summer property. Things had deteriorated to the point that the son and daughter did not want their parents coming over to see the grandchildren.

The psychiatrist told them to let their parents again know how worried they were, that they had come to see him, and that he would be more than willing to meet with them and try to help. The following day, Dr. Smythe called and said, "My wife and I would be delighted to come in, anything to appease the kids, they and the grandchildren mean the world to us." They were a proud and dignified couple, elegantly dressed, formal, and a bit pedantic. Lots of words were spent on their rationalizing and minimizing their use of alcohol, describing their children as "worry warts," and blaming their kids' spouses as "teetotalers and very judgmental." They presented a united front.

The psychiatrist made the strategic decision to leave the whole subject and build rapport by asking about other issues. They were very open to returning. As they were leaving, Mrs. Smythe said: "On the way over to your office, we decided to stop drinking completely. If that will pacify Bob and Paula, then why not? No huge sacrifice on our parts."

They did stop drinking and 11 months later they remained abstinent. Visits focused on classic retirement issues for Dr. Smythe (e.g., need for structure, returning to avocations, taking up new hobbies, and sharing household responsibilities with his wife) and their marriage (e.g., balancing time together and time apart, renewing their sexuality, budgeting on a fixed income, planning travel, and making improvements on their cabin). The psychiatrist found an internist for both of them (for general medical care), and they joined a health club and took up tennis. At the conclusion of treatment, they were doing very well and seemed happy—and so was the extended family.

Although this clinical case report has a happy ending, many couples present far greater resistance to treatment. Often the full complement of addiction treatments is necessary to achieve abstinence.

Making the Diagnosis

Only a portion of physicians who consult their primary care physician or a psychiatrist will include concerns about drinking or drug use in their chief complaint. Asking about substance use is essential in the comprehensive assessment of physicians, both in initial history taking and later if the treating physician has indicators of concern. Many psychiatrists first learn of the possibility of alcohol and other drug use in their physician-patients from concerned family members, who may disclose this information with ambivalence; they are not sure whether it is important or significant. They may worry that their physician loved one is possibly impaired at work, given their use of substances in the evening or on the weekends. They may fear for their wife or husband's medical license and ability to practice. They may worry about repercussions at home, such as anger, rejection, blame, or abandonment, if they report their concerns to a treating health professional.

Symptoms and signs in a physician that are suggestive of substance abuse and dependence have been described by many clinicians. Michael Kaufmann (personal communication, October 2006) emphasizes that the treating clinician must attempt to delineate the performance baseline from which the physician normally functions. He describes early, later, and end-stage signs of addiction:

Early Signs

- Increasingly chaotic lifestyle, financial problems
- More expression of negative thoughts and attitudes
- Increased sensitivity, irritability when approached
- Somatic complaints, illness, and fatigue; "medical" problems
- Withdrawal from friends and family
- Family tension, conflict, infidelity
- Less care in dressing and grooming
- Declining reliability
- Emergence of unhealthy coping behaviors
- Change of work habits, including more time at work

Later Signs

- Angry outbursts at work
- Patient and staff complaints
- Professional withdrawal, deterioration of collegial relationships
- Cancelled clinics and increased absenteeism
- Deterioration of clinical skills and record keeping
- Inappropriate drug handling and diversion
- Alcohol on the breath at work
- Charges of driving under the influence or other offenses
- Family violence, separation, and divorce

End-Stage Signs

- Intoxication at work
- Appearance of chronic illness
- Therapeutic error or mishap
- Extreme personal isolation
- Quitting medicine
- Suicidal gesture
- Suicide

End-stage signs are particularly troubling and highlight the importance of prevention at primary, secondary, and tertiary levels.

Most physician-patients who acknowledge their family's concerns will minimize the true amount of drug that is consumed. In this way, physicians are no different than laypersons with addiction. Taking a detailed history of alcohol and other substance use will help to make the diagnosis or rule it out. Both the content of the answers to one's questions and the attitude and manner of the patient (defensive, guarded, evasive, tending to rationalize) can be illuminating. Commonly used screening instruments are the four-question CAGE questionnaire (Mayfield et al. 1974), the Michigan Alcohol Screening Test (Allen and Columbus 1995), the Alcohol Use Disorders Identification Test (Allen et al. 1997) and the Drug Abuse Screening Test (Skinner 1982). Greenfield and Hennessy's (2004) book chapter on assessment of patients for substance use disorders is an excellent resource. The information is easily applicable to conducting a comprehensive evaluation of an addicted physician. In addition, as we suggested in Chapter 3, collateral information from colleagues and family members is essential.

Most contemporary primary care physicians and psychiatrists are not officially trained in addiction medicine. Once an assessment has been completed and there is a strong suspicion of a substance use disorder, it is prudent to refer the physician-patient to someone who has completed continuing medical education in addictions and is certified by the American Society of Addiction Medicine. This person will not only provide a definitive diagnosis but also outline the best treatment plan. Referral to a certified specialist also serves another purpose. When physician-patients deny or minimize their illness, they are reluctant to accept the opinion of a generalist and often attempt to discredit the credentials of that person. It is harder for them to do this when they have received a thorough assessment by a subspecialist in addiction medicine.

Issues in Treatment

The prognosis for physicians in active practice diagnosed with a substance use disorder is very good. One study reports that at the end of 5 years, 92% of the doctors were drug free and back at work (cited in Adams 2001). Because most physicians who are monitored by state or provincial physician health programs are not self-referred, an intervention may be necessary (Knight et al. 2002). Interventions take many forms, but the general principles outlined and used by the Massachusetts Physician Health Services, including an easy to remember acronym FRAMER (Table 5–1), are a good example (Knight 2004).

It must be emphasized that many interventions are lifesaving. In other words, the impaired physician is so ill and is employing such denial that he or she is completely unable to recognize the illness and seek help. The approach is confrontational but not punitive. The purpose is advocacy. When possible, the intervention team should include recovering physicians as well as peers and family members (Verghese 2002).

Upon completion of the intervention, individuals may receive a comprehensive assessment by a certified addiction medicine specialist. Recommendations are usually made for outpatient or inpatient treatment. With regard to the former, these are usually physicians with at least some acceptance of their illness and willingness to commit to a structured and prescribed program. Physicians with very serious alcohol and drug dependence (especially ones with a lot of denial and outrage at the diagnosis) or physicians who have attempted ambulatory care in the past with one or more relapses are generally referred to a residential treatment center. With this group, rigorous medical and intake investigations are usually completed over the first few days while the physician is being observed and treated for possible alcohol and other drug withdrawal symptoms. This period is followed by several weeks (ranging from 4–12 weeks) of therapy—mostly group treatment but also some individual therapy. The philosophy of most centers is based on the 12-Step approach of Alcoholics Anonymous. Individuals attend daily meetings based on those principles. When a concurrent nonchemical psychiatric illness is present, or detected in recovery, psychiatric consultation with appropriate psychotropic medication is instituted. Physicians may respond better to treatment when referred to residential centers that specialize in treating doctors and other health professionals. Even when these programs are at some geographical distance from where the physician lives or works, spouses, partners, and children should be included as part of the treatment program and provided with information about addictions. On-site couples and family therapy may begin, and it should be recommended that physicians' family members attend Al-Anon, Narconon, Alateen, and other similar groups upon returning home.

A monitored follow-up program is essential in the treatment of addicted doctors to maintain recovery and prevent relapse. Detailed recommendations from the treatment center go to whomever made the referral (e.g., physician health program, primary care physician, medical licensing board) and to all caregivers involved in the ongoing treatment of the physician. This list may include the

TABLE 5–1. Principles of directive interventions: FRAMER

F   Gather all of the FACTS.

R   Determine your RESPONSIBILITY for reporting; consult confidentially with medical and legal experts.

A   Bring in ANOTHER PERSON.

M Begin the meeting with a MONOLOGUE in which you present the facts and summarize your responsibility.

E   Insist on a comprehensive EVALUATION. Refrain from giving a diagnosis.

R   Insist on a REPORT BACK and signed releases allowing all parties to freely communicate.

Source. Adapted with permission from Physician Health Services. A modified version is also available on the Massachusetts Medical Society Web site: www.physicianhealth.org.

physician health program; the addiction medicine specialist who sets up random urine drug screening and regular 1:1 sessions; the Caduceus group leader (often the addiction medicine specialist); the primary care physician; the treating psychiatrist; and any and all psychotherapists providing individual, couples, or family therapy. Caduceus (named after the staff of Asclepius, the Greek god of healing) groups are an important ongoing source of support for a range of health professionals (not just physicians) in recovery. The atmosphere is one of trust, acceptance, mutual caring, and accountability.

Most of the caregivers will be required to submit periodic health updates to the physician health program or directly to the doctor's medical licensing board for a period of time (usually around 5 years). These letters typically address frequency of visits, mood and behavioral stability, safety and competence in the medical workplace (when the physician has returned to work), compliance with prescribed medications, attendance at meetings, and any relapse behavior. The physician being monitored will have signed an agreement or contingency contract with the physician health program or the licensing board that lays out expectations and consequences of noncompliance.

Nonchemical Addictions

An emerging issue in physician health, as elsewhere, is addictive behavior that does not involve use of substances. This problematic behavior may stand alone as a separate diagnosis or it may coexist with a substance use disorder. Examples include pathological gambling, sexual addiction, Internet addiction (or cyberaddiction), compulsive shopping, and exercise addiction. With the exception of pathological gambling, which is listed in DSM-IV-TR (American Psychiatric Association 2000b) under the "impulse-control disorders not elsewhere classified," strict criteria for nonchemical addictions have not been delineated at this time. Are they addictive disorders? Impulse-control disorders? Obsessive-compulsive spectrum disorders? What all of the disorders seem to have in common are

- Continued engagement in the behavior despite adverse consequences to the person's work security, financial stability, marital function, relationship with children, and so forth.
- An inability to stop the behavior, despite protests from the individual that he or she has not lost control.
- Mental preoccupation with the behavior that interferes with the individual's ability to concentrate or attend to work, family, and social life.

No epidemiological data have documented the incidence or prevalence of these disorders in the general population, let alone in physicians. However, physician health programs across North America and mental health professionals who treat doctors describe referrals of physicians with nonchemical addictions. Here are three examples:

Case Examples

Dr. Ames is a 40-year-old family physician who was referred to a psychiatrist by his attorney. He had been suspended from practicing medicine after exposing himself to a woman in the parking lot of his office building. When the woman screamed in horror and ran into an adjoining convenience store for help, Dr. Ames sat in his parked car sobbing until the police came. He was arrested and later released on his own recognizance. On history taking, the psychiatrist learned that Dr. Ames worked in a very busy clinic that had lost two physicians over the previous year. This had resulted in his working harder than usual—essentially 14 hours a day, 6 days a week. His wife and children reacted by coping without him, which ironically compounded his sense of isolation. A pattern developed of arriving home about 9 P.M., giving cursory greetings to his family, and warming up his prepared dinner in the microwave. He then excused himself to dictate his medical charts in his basement office. He would go online and watch pornography with increasing frequency and for longer and longer periods of time, often not going up to bed until 1 or 2 in the morning. "I not only got aroused and got adrenaline pumping, I got obsessed. Like I used to when I was studying for exams in medical school. I got compulsive about having to watch every DVD that a particular porn star was in. I developed an elaborate filing system on my hard drive so that each star was downloaded and stored in alphabetical order. It was weird, just like I had to file my books by author and title on my shelves and my lecture notes in my filing cabinet. I couldn't stop myself, so everything took longer and longer to complete before I could allow myself to go upstairs and get into bed. That day in the parking lot…pulling out my penis…I was ready to burst with overwork and loneliness…. I was out of control…. I wasn't wanting sex with her…. I don't know what I wanted…it all happened so fast…. I didn't even think how terrified she might be of this crazy lunatic…it was like a nervous breakdown…sort of a cry for help."

Dr. Smith is a 34-year-old ophthalmologist who began treatment with her psychiatrist for ongoing management of her major depressive disorder. She was new to the city, but she had been diagnosed with depression during medical school in another state. She had now completed her residency and had started her first job as an attending physician. Her mood was largely stable because of combination antidepressant treatment (bupropion and citalopram) and regular supportive psychotherapy by a psychologist whom she saw during medical school and residency. Dr. Smith was concerned about another problem, however. "I've become a compulsive shopper," she stated. What she described was a pattern of stopping at women's shops and department stores almost every day after work and on weekends. She lived and worked downtown, where shops were within blocks of both locations. Her credit card statement was close to $4,000 monthly, which she paid in full each month. She bought many items of clothing that she never wore. "There are only so many days in a week…. I can't possibly wear all of the dresses, blouses, sweaters, and shoes that I own. I have more makeup than most theater companies have for all of their actors." Dr. Smith had done some thinking about the origins of her compulsive shopping: "I thought at first that I was no different than most women who love to shop, especially for shoes. Is it because I'm done with my residency now and I'm making decent money so that I can afford a nice wardrobe? I know I'm lonely. I don't have a boyfriend. And my self-esteem has never been that terrific. Am I trying to make myself feel better by these little indulgences? My best friend, another doctor, is really worried about me. She thinks I've got an addiction. Maybe she's right. A month ago I tried to stop shopping. I only lasted 3 days. My best friend's a psychiatrist, so she wonders if I'm a little high—maybe my depression is becoming a bipolar disorder."

Dr. Green is a 61-year-old pathologist who was referred to a psychiatrist by his wife, who was worried about him. In his first appointment, Dr. Green presented himself with the following rationalization: "My wife thinks that I have a gambling addiction. I don't agree, but I'll let you be the judge so this doesn't come between my wife and me. We have a wonderful marriage—now in its 36th year." Dr. Green continued: "I like to go to the casino in our city. It's fun and I enjoy the atmosphere. I like consorting with people who I don't see at work or socially. Blackjack is my sport. I'm getting better and better at it. It won't be long before I really hit it big and I can retire from medicine." When the psychiatrist asked him to explain what he meant by "hitting it big," he gave an erudite and excessively detailed lecture on mathematical probabilities about gambling in general and blackjack in particular. Dr. Green denied that he was preoccupied with thoughts about gambling, although his wife found him inaccessible at home, often because of being tied up on the computer. Because of increasing amounts of money spent gambling, Dr. Green did acknowledge that he had tried to quit before but "my heart wasn't in quitting, I only stayed away from the casino to please my wife." He began lying that he was working late at the hospital doing research. When asked if he felt restless or depressed when he was not gambling, he denied any feelings except fraudulence. He said "Why quit something that you love just to keep the peace at home?" When the psychiatrist asked if he was worried about the large amount of money lost, he replied "You would think that would be a wakeup call, wouldn't you? But not for me. That's my incentive to study harder and practice new techniques at the casino. I call it learning 'in situ.' I was taught in medical school and residency that we learn from our mistakes."

One can see from these three examples how critical it is to conduct a thorough and dynamically oriented biopsychosocial assessment of physicians presenting with nonchemical addictive behavior. Because the physician's insight may be minimal to absent, interviewing family members and/or concerned work colleagues may be essential. Rationalization and denial are common defenses in physicians with these disorders; many of them cannot grasp how much the behavior has taken over their lives or appreciate the serious consequences of their actions. Moreover, physicians with addictions may be unaware of how their behavior is affecting those who live and work with them. These conditions may overlap with impulse-control disorders, sexual disorders, personality disorders, and bipolar illness.

Rather than attempt to discuss all of the various nonchemical addictions that might affect physicians, we focus only on sexual addiction. This is not because of its prevalence, but because it is probably the most upsetting (and shameful) for the physician and for his family and colleagues. In addition, if the sexual behavior involves professional boundary violations, serious harm can be done to patients, coworkers, and the profession itself. Boundary violations are considered in greater detail in Chapter 7.

Compulsive Sexual Behavior or Sexual Addiction

Fong (2006) noted that the lack of formalized criteria for compulsive sexual behavior can be explained in part by the lack of research and an agreed-upon terminology and the heterogeneous presentation of compulsive sexual behaviors. Some patients have symptoms that resemble an addictive disorder—for example, continued engagement in the behavior despite physical and psychological consequences, loss of control, and preoccupation with the action. Other symptoms are more like those of impulse-control disorders—strong and irresistible urges, both physically and mentally, to act out sexually without regard to consequences. Some forms of sexual addiction are confused with OCD. Indeed, physicians who are overtaken by sexual impulses may actually prefer to think of themselves as having OCD, a biologically based disorder that relieves them of a sense of personal responsibility for their behavior. However, OCD is characterized by ego-dystonic rituals that are NOT pleasant. Behaviors that feel good are not characteristic of OCD.

Of the two categories of compulsive sexual behavior (Fong 2006)—paraphilic and nonparaphilic—the vast majority of physicians with this diagnosis are in the second group. These are doctors with addiction to pornography, visiting prostitutes, going to strip bars and clubs, cruising (in gay and bisexual physicians), and extramarital relationships. The clinician must carefully assess the patient to clarify whether the behavior indeed shows a compulsive or addictive pattern—in effect, is it time-consuming and intruding on the doctor's professional or personal life? Nonparaphilic compulsive behavior must be distinguished from sexual behaviors that have other sources and are not truly addictive:

- *Situational.* In this case, the physician only views pornography or goes to strip clubs when he or she is lonely. A rural physician, for example, may attend a medical conference in a large urban center and visit a gentlemen's club. Other physicians may be bored or tired and log on to a hospital computer during a slow night of in-house call. Still other physicians may resort to sexual behavior to soothe anxiety. For example, a cardiac surgeon who cannot sleep prior to a complicated procedure the following morning may engage in masturbatory behavior while viewing an adult magazine.
- *Marital (or other intimate relationship) problem.* Unhappy in his marriage, the physician seeks sexual gratification or some other type of intimacy by hiring an escort or prostitute. A conflicted married bisexual physician may have periodic furtive and impersonal sexual experiences with people contacted via the Internet or gay newspapers.
- *Unrecognized or untreated mood disorder.* Both depressed and hypomanic physicians may have sexual symptoms. The behavior is usually ego-dystonic and is related to a dysphoric or elevated mood. In depression, watching pornographic movies temporarily lifts the person's mood. In hypomania, picking up a prostitute is a result of disinhibition and heightened libido.

The interface of narcissistic and borderline personality disorders (see Chapter 6) with sexual addictions is complicated. Many male heterosexual physicians, for example, will claim to have a sex addiction. However, when they undergo a thorough psychiatric evaluation, they reveal a view of women as degraded and objectified sexual playthings. They have little or no remorse for the emotional pain they cause women and little empathy for the female partner's internal subjective struggles involved with the sexual relationship. Women in relationships with them feel used and discarded.

Another complication in the use of the term *sex addiction* is that it can be applied in a pejorative, moralizing sense. Human sexual behavior takes many forms, and a nonjudgmental tolerance is an essential quality for physicians and other healthcare professionals in their approach to patients. When one evaluates a physician's sexuality, one must consider whether the sexual behavior truly causes problems in social or occupational functioning or is simply different than mainstream sexual behavior as defined by the predominant cultural standards.

Issues in Treatment of Nonchemical Addictions

There are many principles in the management of substance use disorders that are applicable in the treatment of nonchemical addictions in physicians. Once a diagnosis is made, biopsychosocial considerations are in order. Pharmacotherapy may be indicated. Selective serotonin reuptake inhibitors may be helpful, usually in higher dosages than are used in the treatment of depression (Bradford 2001), but more data from rigorously controlled trials are needed to recommend these agents with a high degree of confidence. Clomipramine has also been used with some success. In a recent study of pathological gamblers (Grant et al. 2006), the opioid antagonist nalmefene at a low dosage of 25 mg/day was found to be efficacious in reducing the severity of symptoms. Sexual impulses and arousal have been reduced with naltrexone (Ryback 2004). In general, mood stabilizers have been helpful only when there is a concurrent diagnosis of bipolar mood disorder. Anti-androgens have been used to treat severe sexual addictions and paraphilias with some degree of success.

There are many psychosocial approaches to nonchemical addictions in physicians. Gamblers Anonymous and Sexaholics Anonymous, both modeled on 12-Step principles, are the mainstays for gambling and sexual addictions. Residential treatment centers exist for the assessment and treatment of individuals with compulsive sexual disorders and other nonchemical addictions. The basics include education, individual and group counseling, spiritual exercises, and family therapy. Cognitive-behavioral therapy is very helpful for patients to identify what triggers their repetitive behavior, what reinforces it, and what thought techniques can be implemented to prevent their habitual actions. Psychodynamically oriented psychotherapy may be useful for some physicians with histories of abuse, loss, poor self-esteem, sexual conflict, and impulsivity. Marital, family, and group therapies are all important modalities of treatment for physicians whose addictions have affected intimacy, homeostasis, trust, and connection.

Despite growing experience with the treatment of nonchemical addictions, the field remains in its infancy. Much has yet to be learned about what works and what is ineffective. Few randomized, controlled trials exist to guide clinicians. Some forms of addictive behavior present special challenges. Cyberaddiction, for example, poses a problem in finding an analogy to abstinence from the substance abuse model. Computers are an essential feature of modern life. Asking a physician to abstain from computer use is not reasonable, and restricting the use to optimal levels and appropriate professional uses is not easily enforced. Hence a good deal of the treatment for nonchemical addictions involves guesswork, clinical wisdom, and trial and error.

Future Directions

The assessment and treatment of addicted physicians is ever evolving. In a recent and evocative paper that addresses performance failures in physicians, Leape and Fromson (2006) decry the shortcomings of the methods currently in place to ensure the quality and safety of a physician's work. They call for a national effort and urge the Federation of State Medical Boards, the American Board of Medical Specialties, and the Joint Commission on Accreditation of Healthcare Organizations to collaborate on developing better methods for measuring performance and to expand programs for helping physicians who are deficient. Because drug and alcohol addiction in physicians can, in some cases, result in patient injury, Leape and Fromson see a need for expansion of assessment and remediation programs and recommend implementing annual physical examinations and random drug testing for all physicians. They also raise for discussion the notion of routine cognitive evaluation for older physicians. Their recommendation for random drug testing is supported by Gold and Frost-Pineda (2006): "Although all physicians are at risk and should be monitored, we strongly recommend that priority be given to specialists with greatest access to and greatest risk for occupational exposure (anesthesiologists, surgeons, and emergency medicine specialists)" (p. 861). Substantial numbers of practicing physicians, residency program directors, and medical students oppose such testing (Donohoe 2005).

Not all physicians with addictions will embrace, even over time, a treatment that is rooted in principles of Alcoholics Anonymous. Although 12-Step programs have been the gold standard of care for addicted physicians, alternative approaches have been proposed. In a study by Warhaft (2006), there was no difference in outcome between two groups of physicians, 12-Step and non-12-Step, at 5 years after recovery. Outcomes were based on relapses, deaths, and capacity to resume medical practice. Although the author does not present details of the non-12-Step approaches, they are designed on a case by case basis and are described as "high quality, intense, and enduring." Motivational enhancement and cognitive-behavioral therapies have been found to be effective in some groups but to our knowledge have not been studied in physicians specifically (see Chapter 9). Given the number of addicted physicians who avoid 12-Step programs or who drop out and are at risk of increased morbidity and dying of their disease, evidence-based research in alternative therapies is essential.

Key Points

- Both chemical (substance use disorders) and nonchemical (non–substance use disorders) addictions occur in physicians. The estimated lifetime incidence of substance use disorders in physicians is 8%–15%. The incidence of nonchemical addictions in physicians is unknown.

- In addition to genetic vulnerability to addictions, physicians are subject to other determinants. These include a knowledge about and openness to the use of pharmacological agents, an intellectual tendency to argue against susceptibility in oneself, strong will and determination, experimentation with drugs, and a predisposition to overwork and justification of chemical relief.

- Because many addicted physicians do not seek help voluntarily, interventions are often necessary. Basic principles have been worked out over the years and should be followed by physician health programs and hospital committees.

- Both chemical and nonchemical addictions have biopsychosocial underpinnings. Thorough and comprehensive assessment and treatment by a team of health professionals are usually necessary and ensure compliance and recovery.

- Many physicians with addictions also have concurrent psychiatric disorders (mood disorders, anxiety disorders, eating disorders, and personality disorders). It is imperative that these illnesses receive attention and that psychiatrists work closely with addiction medicine specialists to be clear about treatment goals and to foster mutual respect.

- Untreated chemical and nonchemical addictions are serious. They adversely affect every dimension of the lives of physicians—their physical, mental, and spiritual health; marriage; relationships with children; work colleagues; and ability to practice medicine. Suicide is the most tragic outcome.

- The prognosis for recovery in physicians is excellent, with more than 90% of practicing physicians working again at 5 years.

Personality Disorders, Personality Traits, and Disruptive Physicians

Physician health programs were born out of concern that addicted physicians were destroying themselves and jeopardizing the safety of their patients. Over time the addiction perspective has broadened to include depression, dementia, and other psychiatric conditions. In recent years there has been a growing interest in the "disruptive physician." This designation is often a euphemism for describing personality disordered behavior in physicians. Behaviors vary widely but may include explosions of anger, lack of professionalism in the way that one treats colleagues or patients, divisiveness in working with hospital administration or members of one's group, gossiping in public about colleagues, using obscenities in the workplace, making sexually or racially insensitive comments, arrogance, refusing to follow regulations, failing to complete paperwork or respond to pages, being impulsive, and engaging in corrupt practices. Many of these behaviors cannot be explained by an Axis I psychiatric condition and instead involve long-standing patterns of maladaptive behavior and thinking that create chronic problems in the workplace and in relationships (both personal and professional).

The approach to the diagnosis of physicians typically emphasizes Axis I syndromes, with a relative neglect of the role of personality problems in the pathogenesis and maintenance of these symptomatic behaviors. Many symptoms of personality disorders are ego-syntonic, meaning that they do not cause distress in the patient, but, rather, they cause distress in others. Hence such physicians may not seek help for their problematic behaviors in the workplace. They may maintain that that is the way they are and that they are not interested in changing. In some cases, the physician may be technically competent, or even outstanding, but profoundly irritating to colleagues, coworkers, and patients.

Case Example

A 50-year-old primary care practitioner, Dr. Hardesty, had a complaint filed against him by a female patient who reported that he had walked into the examination room and exclaimed, "You smell like a French whore!" She was deeply offended by his comment. When Dr. Hardesty was evaluated at the request of the licensing board, his evaluating clinician asked him why he had made such a hurtful comment to a patient. He replied, "Because I tell the truth. That's what my patients like about me. I'm honest! She DID smell like a French whore. I was in France in my youth, and I know what they smell like." He was utterly unrepentant for his breach of professionalism and was not able to see that his behavior was a problem.

Not all personality disorders manifest themselves in disruptive behaviors. Some, like obsessive-compulsive personality disorder (OCPD), involve heightened conscientiousness and overwork, leading to burnout and depression. These traits are an extreme version of the compulsiveness and perfectionism described in Chapter 1 ("The Psychology of Physicians and the Culture of Medicine") that are commonly found in most physicians.

DSM-IV-TR (American Psychiatric Association 2000b) describes 10 personality disorders and divides them into three clusters: Cluster A, the eccentric cluster; Cluster B, the dramatic cluster; and Cluster C, the anxious cluster. Although this classification is helpful, physicians often manifest mixtures of symptoms from different personality disorders, leading to a diagnosis of personality disorder not otherwise specified, often referred to as "mixed" personality disorder. Indeed, this diagnostic wastebasket may be the most common personality disorder diagnosed when assessing physicians. Table 6–1 lists all 10 personality disorders, but in this chapter, because of space limitations, we limit ourselves to three common entities seen in the evaluation of physicians: narcissistic, borderline, and obsessive-compulsive. Moreover, there are many instances in which physicians may be disruptive, but they do not meet diagnostic criteria for a personality disorder. Personality traits that fall short of the threshold for an Axis II diagnosis may still create problems in the workplace.

Before concluding that personality traits or a personality disorder is the primary cause of the disruptive behavior, an evaluating clinician must rule out other causes of the behavior, such as alcohol or drug abuse, bipolar illness, or a neurological process. Collateral information from colleagues and family members may

TABLE 6–1. DSM-IV-TR personality disorders

Cluster A
    Paranoid
    Schizoid
    Schizotypal
Cluster B
    Borderline
    Narcissistic
    Histrionic
    Antisocial
Cluster C
    Obsessive-Compulsive
    Avoidant
    Dependent

be extremely helpful in making these distinctions. Urine drug screenings are useful in detecting drug or alcohol problems. Neuropsychological testing is essential for diagnosing early signs of dementia or frontal lobe disturbances stemming from other causes. One must also keep in mind the possibility that comorbidity involving *both* an Axis II personality disorder and an Axis I syndrome, such as depression, bipolar illness, or chemical dependency, is responsible for the clinical picture. Multiple conditions complicate the treatment planning and generally make the prognosis a bit more guarded. In any case, in this chapter we consider the common personality disorders as entities in their own right.

Narcissistic Personality Disorder

Physicians are often referred to as having a "God complex" and may be regarded as arrogant or self-absorbed in their style of relating to others. An old joke captures this image: A newly deceased applicant to heaven appears at the pearly gates. He notes a man in a white coat with a stethoscope around his neck and asks St. Peter, "Do you have doctors here?" St. Peter retorts, "No, no. That's God. He just likes to play doctor from time to time."

The DSM-IV-TR criteria for narcissistic personality disorder are listed in Table 6–2. These criteria, although useful, do not capture the fundamental insecurity in narcissistic individuals, who may relate to others with bluster or bravado to mask their own self-doubt. Narcissism is reflective of problematic self-development involving a lack of self-esteem and self-coherence. These individuals may be desperately seeking validation, affirmation, and approval from others as a way to shore up their shaky sense of self-confidence. Beneath the arrogant surface is a needy child yearning to be loved, respected, and regarded as competent. As with most personality disorders, the cause of the condition is not clear, but the pathogenesis probably involves a genetically based temperament acted on by environmental stressors early in life (Gabbard 2005a).

Case Example

Dr. Sims was a 58-year-old general surgeon who created problems in the operating room, in medical staff meetings, in grand rounds, and in his office. He was regarded as a know-it-all by his peers, and his displays of self-aggrandizement and contempt toward others were legendary in the hospital. In the middle of a grand rounds presentation on a case of a gastrointestinal hemorrhage, a colleague from the medicine department was describing how he used endoscopic techniques to diagnosis the origin of the bleeding. Dr. Sims interrupted him from the audience, stood up, and launched into a tirade: "Why on earth waste time with endoscopy? You know there's a bleed and you know you're gonna have to operate. Why not just open the patient up and repair the bleed? This kind of presentation is a frequent problem in these rounds. We bring in colleagues outside of the surgery department who tell us about the latest fiber optic device as though it really adds something to what we do. I've been operating for 30 years and I don't need to be told what to do. What a colossal waste of time!" At this point Dr. Sims stomped out of the auditorium. His colleagues shook their heads, and one said to another under his breath, "That's Sims for you!"

Dr. Sims yelled at nurses and operating room technicians during surgical procedures and lost his temper with his office employees as well. During an operation, he would humiliate medical students. For example, during a surgical procedure, he would typically ask the student observing the procedure if he could point out the foramen of Winslow. If the student failed to answer the question correctly, he would make disparaging comments like, "Oh, I forgot. Your generation doesn't read. They just watch MTV and play computer games." If a student wasn't adequately prepared when presenting a patient to Dr. Sims on service rounds, he would berate the student. He said to one student, "How dare you waste the time of an attending, one resident, one intern, and three other students by coming to rounds unprepared!" The chief of the medical staff of his teaching hospital said that complaints had accumulated for many years, but the hospital had not acted on them because Dr. Sims was an excellent surgeon and brought in a good deal of business. His colleagues regarded him as unable to alter his behavior and simply tolerated him, avoiding interaction with him whenever possible. The chief of staff also noted that his behavior had recently become worse, and he wondered if Dr. Sims was experiencing something in his personal life that was exacerbating his longstanding personality traits. He said that recent complaints included instances where he had reduced medical students and nurses to tears by his insensitive comments. The chief of staff also stated emphatically that drug or alcohol abuse had never been implicated, and Dr. Sims's wife subsequently corroborated that Dr. Sims rarely drank and did not use controlled substances.

When he arrived for evaluation, Dr. Sims made it clear that he regarded himself as a scapegoat and was disgruntled about being sent for an assessment.

TABLE 6–2.   DSM-IV-TR criteria for narcissistic personality disorder

A pervasive pattern of grandiosity (in fantasy or behavior), need for admiration, and lack of empathy, beginning by early adulthood and present in a variety of contexts, as indicated by five (or more) of the following:

1)   Has a grandiose sense of self-importance (e.g., exaggerates achievements and talents, expects to be recognized as superior without commensurate achievements)

2)   Is preoccupied with fantasies of unlimited success, power, brilliance, beauty, or ideal love

3)   Believes that he or she is "special" and unique and can only be understood by, or should associate with, other special or high-status people (or institutions)

4)   Requires excessive admiration

5)   Has a sense of entitlement, i.e., unreasonable expectations of especially favorable treatment or automatic compliance with his or her expectations

6)   Is interpersonally exploitative, i.e., takes advantage of others to achieve his or her own ends

7)   Lacks empathy: is unwilling to recognize or identify with the feelings and needs of others

8)   Is often envious of others or believes that others are envious of him or her

9)   Shows arrogant, haughty behaviors or attitudes

He claimed that he was the focus of envy by those who were not as successful as he was. His evaluator asked him about the contempt he displayed toward others and his public humiliation of students and coworkers. He responded that these complaints were greatly exaggerated. He said that he was personally responsible for many students entering surgery as a specialty. He retorted, "I've taught hundreds of medical students, and only two or three complained. That should make you wonder how representative these complaints are." He also elaborated at great length about how badly *he* was treated when he was in training, and said, "If you can't stand the heat, get out of the kitchen." When the evaluator allowed him time to ramble a bit, Dr. Sims revealed how frustrated he was with the way medicine as a profession was going. He said he was feeling increasingly irrelevant, because students today had a different set of values. He thought the limitation on work hours for residents was absurd and that too many students whined and complained about having to work. He clearly felt his power and influence were beginning to wane. As he continued to talk, he made several references to the past, when he was a "handsome, dashing figure" whom female nurses wanted to date. The evaluator began to discern that aging itself was a narcissistic injury for Dr. Sims, who was struggling with a crisis of adult development on top of his longstanding narcissistic personality disorder. The arrogance viewed by others appeared to be a defense against his feeling of insecurity that he no longer was seen as the powerful and sexually desirable heroic figure that he once was.

The case of Dr. Sims illustrates a frequent problem in narcissistic and disruptive physicians. Their insensitivity and lack of empathy reflects a deficit in the capacity to *mentalize*. The concept of *mentalization* has emerged from attachment theory and has received empirical support from a growing body of research (Fonagy and Target 2001). It refers to the capacity to understand that one's own and others' thinking is representational in nature and that one's own and others' behavior is motivated by internal states, such as thoughts and feelings. The ability to mentalize is often referred to as having a "theory of mind." In other words, one is aware that each person has a separate subjectivity based on life experience that creates a unique mind. Experience is filtered through this mind.

Insecure attachment linked to childhood trauma may, in some individuals with personality disorders, interfere with the capacity to mentalize (Fonagy and Target 2001). As a result, physicians with this difficulty cannot place themselves in the minds of others and understand how their comments affect those around them. In addition, they fail to see that their own views are simply one perspective based on their own feelings, beliefs, and biases. They assume that their point of view is the definitive truth and that others are misguided. They also cannot understand how others misconstrue what they say. In Dr. Sims's view, he was trying to teach students and nurses how to do things the "right way." From their standpoint, he was humiliating them. He could not see that his intent was not the same as the impact he had on others. Hence he was oblivious to how he affected others and could not see the problem that he was creating in the workplace. When the evaluator explained to Dr. Sims that this was a problem in professionalism rather than in his competence as a surgeon, Dr. Sims replied, "Don't tell me what's professional. I wrote the book on that."

His response was an example of a related problem—poor judgment in his interpersonal relations. Because of his problems in mentalizing, he could not accurately anticipate the consequences of his actions, so he was repeatedly offending others and shooting himself in the foot with his choices. He had few friends and a wife who felt their marriage was dead. When she was interviewed by the social worker on the team, she said that her husband was a dedicated surgeon but that their marriage was only a "marriage of convenience" at this point.

Dr. Sims also illustrates one of the major problems with people who have narcissistic personality disorders—they age terribly. The loss of physical attractiveness, sexual prowess, and respect from others makes them feel even more insecure than before. Their envy makes it difficult for them to enjoy the success of those in the next generation and take pleasure in mentoring them (Gabbard 2005b). They grow old, bitter, and resentful and may take out their bitterness on those in their surroundings.

Narcissistic personality disorder is difficult to treat, especially when the physician diagnosed with the condition is not motivated to seek help or change. We have no randomized controlled trials involving treatment of this disorder, and the outcome is uncertain. Similarly, there are no long-term follow-up studies on disruptive physicians who fit this profile. In the case of Dr. Sims, the evaluating team wrote a report that was sent to the chief of the medical staff who had made th referral and to Dr. Sims himself. The report diagnosed narcissistic personality disorder and described his problems with mentalization and judgment. It also clarified that he was not impaired to practice but had serious problems in professionalism. The following recommendations were made:

1. Psychotherapy to learn greater self-reflection and to increase his capacity to mentalize about others' experience of him. The therapy could also address his crisis of adult development and help him mourn the loss of his youth. The psychotherapist only had to report that Dr. Sims attended the sessions, not the content, so as to preserve confidentiality.
2. A continuing education seminar on professionalism so Dr. Sims could be brought up to date on how times have changed and how behaviors that were once tolerated are no longer acceptable.
3. A form of monitoring known as "360-degree monitoring." In other words, those who worked with him in the operating room, on ward rounds, and in education had a checklist of problematic behaviors that they would fill out each month and turn in to the chief of the medical staff, who would then go over the reports with Dr. Sims. In this way, he was receiving feedback (anonymously) on a regular basis and had to improve on his obliviousness by considering how others were reacting to him.
4. An agreement that Dr. Sims would be given a 6-month trial of this treatment plan with a reconsideration of whether it was working at the end of that time period. If this plan failed, termination of his privileges at the hospital would be considered. This last measure put "teeth" into the plan so that Dr. Sims knew there were serious consequences for his actions.

The treatment plan should in no way preempt appropriate disciplinary action from the hospital (or licensing board). The clinical assessment and the adjudication of misconduct must operate independently. Indeed, if the physician transgresses hospital policy during the period of rehabilitation, he or she must face the consequences.

Even with a comprehensive treatment plan, disruptive physicians with narcissistic personality disorder may not improve with treatment. They may reluctantly go along with treatment because they feel coerced. They may show up at psychotherapy sessions but have nothing to say. They may use the psychotherapy to complain about how they have been treated. In Chapter 8 ("Psychodynamic Psychotherapy") we discuss the technique of dynamic psychotherapy with these patients in more detail. Suffice it to say, however, that they may not be responsive to any treatment approach and may end up resigning their privileges to avoid the narcissistic injury of being dismissed. They may also move elsewhere, thinking that a geographic move will change their internal world.

Another variant on narcissistic personality disorder is a malignant subtype with antisocial features. It is rather unusual to see a physician in practice who meets DSM-IV-TR criteria for antisocial personality disorder. These criteria are weighted in the direction of criminal behavior, and most physicians would have been drummed out of the profession at some point in training if they met these criteria. However, one regularly finds corrupt or antisocial features in narcissistic personality disorders (Gabbard 2005b; Kernberg 1984), and when physicians have these features, the public may be in grave danger. Such physicians may have lied, cheated on examinations, and falsified medical records in the course of their education and eluded detection. Others may have been caught but threatened to sue the medical school or residency if they were to be dismissed from their program. These threats may have intimidated faculty committees, who then chose not to pursue disciplinary actions. Such physicians may come to light in a number of ways—Medicare or insurance fraud, sexual misconduct with patients, callousness in their interactions with patients, lying about mistakes they have made, or supplying drugs to drug-seeking individuals.

Physicians who come for evaluation with these accusations may be challenging to assess. They may adamantly deny the charges and make the evaluator feel cruel and sadistic for agreeing with external parties who feel that corrupt practices are an issue. Some narcissistically organized individuals can be extraordinarily charming and convince the evaluating clinician that a grave injustice has been done to them. Collateral sources become of paramount importance in such evaluations, and the evaluating team must be diligent in collecting those sources prior to seeing the patient. Those physicians who have this alarming degree of corruption and lack of remorse should not be treated or rehabilitated. They are unlikely to benefit from treatment and will very likely return to their corrupt practices. They need to be redirected into other lines of work.

Borderline Personality Disorder

Like narcissistic personality disorder, borderline personality disorder (BPD) is one of the dramatic, or Cluster B, entities that can lead to highly disruptive behavior. The physician with BPD is likely to be more erratic in his or her behavior

TABLE 6–3.   DSM-IV-TR criteria for borderline personality disorder

A pervasive pattern of instability of interpersonal relationships, self-image, and affects, and marked impulsivity beginning by early adulthood and present in a variety of contexts, as indicated by five (or more) of the following:

1) Frantic efforts to avoid real or imagined abandonment. **Note:** Do not include suicidal or self-mutilating behavior covered in Criterion 5.

2) A pattern of unstable and intense interpersonal relationships characterized by alternating between extremes of idealization and devaluation

3) Identity disturbance: markedly and persistently unstable self-image or sense of self

4) Impulsivity in at least two areas that are potentially self-damaging (e.g., spending, sex, substance abuse, reckless driving, binge eating). **Note:** Do not include suicidal or self-mutilating behavior covered in Criterion 5.

5) Recurrent suicidal behavior, gestures, or threats or self-mutilating behavior

6) Affective instability due to a marked reactivity of mood (e.g., intense episodic dysphoria, irritability, or anxiety usually lasting a few hours and only rarely more than a few days)

7) Chronic feelings of emptiness

8) Inappropriate, intense anger or difficulty controlling anger (e.g., frequent displays of temper, constant anger, recurrent physical fights)

9) Transient, stress-related paranoid ideation or severe dissociative symptoms

than physicians with narcissistic personality disorder. As the diagnostic criteria indicate (see Table 6–3), persons with this condition are highly emotional and potentially self-destructive.

Persons with BPD represent a continuum from those with a relatively high-functioning variant to those with a low-functioning subtype that sometimes requires hospitalization. Because only five of the nine criteria are necessary for the diagnosis, some BPD patients with select criteria may manage to gain admission to medical school and succeed in getting through a residency. However, they have generally been noted to have considerable variability in function and to be well regarded by some while seen as problematic by others. Characteristically, they use the defense of splitting in their internal object relations, such that views of the self and other are extreme. Those with whom they are close are either idealized or devalued; thus, the former may view the borderline person positively, whereas the latter may see the person as contemptible.

Physicians with BPD are frequently regarded as potentially explosive because of their intense anger. Others may feel that they have to walk on eggshells around them and make special exceptions for them so as to avoid angry outbursts (Gabbard 2005b). In some cases, self-mutilation or suicide attempts are part of the clinical picture, and these risks make others even more cautious in confronting them about unacceptable behavior in the workplace. As a result, physicians with BPD may get away with things that their colleagues do not.

Some of the physicians with BPD who are in the higher range of the continuum may function reasonably well at work. Others may manifest an underlying fragility and an emotional lability, but they may be intelligent enough to succeed and to render reasonably good patient care. Their personal lives, on the other hand, may be chaotic and a source of great distress. They may go through one relationship after another in which they are rapidly swept off their feet with passion only to be disillusioned and rejected shortly thereafter. This "roller coaster" pattern may influence their attitude at work and make others wonder why they are so "moody" or "unpredictable."

Case Example

Dr. Lewis was a 35-year-old neurologist who had managed to get through medical school and residency successfully with the help of a good deal of psychotherapy. She was regarded as an intelligent and competent neurologist, but she was also viewed as someone who was chronically unhappy. She ran into a number of conflicts with her colleagues over management of patients, and she was known to be volatile. At times she would erupt in rage at colleagues whom she viewed as unfairly criticizing her or questioning her judgment.

Dr. Lewis called and made an appointment to see a psychiatrist on her own because of her repeated frustrations at work and her chronic problems in her personal life. She had had a number of relationships with men whom she retrospectively regarded as "sleazy" and always felt used and discarded by the men she dated. She also said that her female friends became jealous of her because of her intelligence and physical attractiveness and tended to lose interest in their friendship with her. She said she had a difficult time trusting others and often felt lonely and empty as a result. Dr. Lewis noted that she was not really sure who she was and that she showed dramatically different sides of herself to different people. She said that in her previous psychotherapy she had tried to integrate all the different aspects of herself but found it difficult to have a firm sense of identity.

As with many patients who have BPD, Dr. Lewis had a tragic history of childhood trauma. Her mother had divorced her father when Dr. Lewis was only 3 years old, and her stepfather had sexually abused her from the age of 7 to the age of 12, when she threatened to tell her mother if the stepfather did not stop.

She subsequently experienced date rape and had a number of emotionally abusive relationships with men. She often thought of herself as "damaged goods" and felt that no man would ever want to marry her. She frequently described an inner experience of "deadness" and went through many months in which she described no gratification whatsoever in her work. She was chronically suicidal, but she never acted on it because she was Catholic and convinced that she would go to hell if she took her own life.

She felt that psychotherapy had helped in the past, but she said that she had quit prematurely because she could not stand the periods of separation from her psychotherapist. She said she became overly attached and overly dependent on him and had to break off the relationship. She said that she felt toward the therapist as she did with some men with whom she had been involved. She said she would function fine until she got involved with men, and then she would become "crazy," by which she meant being constantly anxious about whether she would be rejected or whether the man with whom she was involved would like another woman better than her. She would become so preoccupied that she would be unable to carry out her responsibilities in a way that felt professional to her. However, no complaints had actually been filed against her.

She told the psychiatrist that she consulted for psychotherapy that she would also like to begin taking a selective serotonin reuptake inhibitor (SSRI) that had been helpful in the past. She said the medication had "evened her out" so that her mood fluctuation was less, and she was able to be more reflective in therapy. She also said that while she was in treatment, she had a place to process what had happened at work so that the slights she felt hurt less and she was able to get along somewhat better with her coworkers and colleagues.

The psychiatrist outlined a treatment plan that involved a totally confidential treatment relationship, including twice-weekly dynamic psychotherapy and the prescription of escitalopram, 20 mg daily. She explained to Dr. Lewis that the treatment would remain confidential, but if she felt that patient care was being jeopardized because of her condition, she would inform Dr. Lewis and consider what measures needed to be taken to protect patient care. Dr. Lewis said she understood and would cooperate with this plan. Her psychiatrist also indicated that confidentiality might have to be broken under circumstances in which she felt there was danger to the self or to others.

Dr. Lewis's BPD represents the high-functioning end of the spectrum. Her distress was sufficient that she sought treatment voluntarily and did not undergo any monitoring by a physicians health program or other external agency. The etiology of BPD is multifactorial and involves such influences as childhood trauma, neglect, genetic predisposition, problematic family dynamics, and neuropsychological difficulties (Gabbard 2005a). It may also involve biological factors, such as a hyperreactive hypothalamic-pituitary-adrenal axis and excessive amygdalar activity. As is often the case, Dr. Lewis reexperienced much of her childhood trauma in her adult relationships. She frequently perceived others as malevolent or attacking her, and she found it extremely difficult to trust. She also dealt with intense separation anxiety and found it difficult to soothe herself and feel stable regarding her own sense of identity. She felt she was always on an emotional roller coaster that made her miserable and suicidal. Frequently in the psychotherapy she told her psychiatrist that her work was what kept her organized and functional and that she was relieved to have a structured workday that she could count on from week to week.

In contrast to narcissistic personality disorder, there are randomized controlled trials showing that psychotherapy can be efficacious with BPD. Several different types of psychotherapy have been shown to be useful, including dialectical behavior therapy (Linehan et al. 1991), mentalization-based therapy (Bateman and Fonagy 1999, 2001), transference-focused therapy (Clarkin et al. 2007), and schema-focused psychotherapy (Giesen-Bloo et al. 2006). Several double-blind, placebo-controlled trials have also demonstrated that SSRIs are useful adjuncts to the psychotherapy of BPD (see Coccaro and Kavoussi 1997; Markovitz 1995; Rinne et al. 2002; Salzman et al. 1995). Research has shown that it takes generally a year or more of treatment for psychotherapy to start showing substantial results and that the treatment must be considered long-term in its duration, as in treatments required for narcissistic personality disorder. Individuals with BPD may be at risk for suicide, and hospitalization is sometimes necessary. The prognosis is generally reasonably good if patients receive the specialized type of treatment necessary. If their functioning is too chaotic, however, they may need to take periods of time off from the practice of medicine until the treatment has restored their functioning to a level that is safe for patient care.

Obsessive-Compulsive Personality Disorder

The traits of OCPD were covered to some extent in Chapter 1, because obsessive-compulsive traits are pervasive in those who become physicians. As noted previously, certain features commonly associated with OCPD are adaptive and lead to success in medical education and the practice of medicine. Perfectionistic tendencies and a thoroughness in everything that one does can lead to efficient and highly competent medical practice. On the other hand, the disorder itself is not likely to be diagnosed unless the individual physician is becoming ineffective and dysfunctional in certain ways. Excessive perfectionism may lead to difficulty in completing one's work and may seriously compromise personal relationships. The diagnostic criteria for OCPD are listed in Table 6–4.

In addition, when excessive feelings of self-doubt, guilt, and responsibility consume the physician, a sense of inner torment can contribute to a lack of fulfillment in one's work. As noted in Chapter 1, physicians in training who perceive that they are making mistakes are more likely to feel a sense of depression, personal distress, and decreased empathy. Indeed, longitudinal follow-up stud-

---

TABLE 6–4. DSM-IV-TR criteria for obsessive-compulsive personality disorder

---

A pervasive pattern of preoccupation with orderliness, perfectionism, and mental and interpersonal control, at the expense of flexibility, openness, and efficiency, beginning by early adulthood and present in a variety of contexts, as indicated by four (or more) of the following:

1) Is preoccupied with details, rules, lists, order, organization, or schedules to the extent that the major point of the activity is lost

2) Shows perfectionism that interferes with task completion (e.g., is unable to complete a project because his or her own overly strict standards are not met)

3) Is excessively devoted to work and productivity to the exclusion of leisure activities and friendships (not accounted for by obvious economic necessity)

4) Is overconscientious, scrupulous, and inflexible about matters of morality, ethics, or values (not accounted for by cultural or religious identification)

5) Is unable to discard worn-out or worthless objects even when they have no sentimental value

6) Is reluctant to delegate tasks or to work with others unless they submit to exactly his or her way of doing things

7) Adopts a miserly spending style toward both self and others; money is viewed as something to be hoarded for future catastrophes

8) Shows rigidity and stubbornness

---

ies of personality disorders (Skodol et al. 1999) indicate that OCPD patients may deteriorate into depression at higher rates than patients with some other personality disorders.

A familiar picture associated with OCPD is the physician who is striving for perfection yet always falling short. These physicians may chastise themselves for not working harder and become increasingly devoted to work and productivity while forgoing any personal life or fun outside of medicine. They become increasingly determined to avoid any type of error and try to control all of those around them so that everything is done in exactly the way they wish it to be done. They may not be disruptive in the way that narcissistic or borderline physicians are, but they annoy and irritate others with their controlling tendencies and their subtle "holier than thou" attitude in their approach to the practice of medicine. This driven, workaholic lifestyle may eventually lead to burnout.

Spickard et al. (2002) have described midcareer burnout and catalogued the typical signs of the syndrome. These include cynicism, a sense of depersonalization at work and in relationships with colleagues, a sense of emotional exhaustion, and perceived clinical ineffectiveness. In addition, fatigue, irritability, sleep problems, headaches, depression, and impaired job performance are all associated with burnout. Such physicians may show up at work every day, but their subjective experience is that of a modern-day Sisyphus who pushes the boulder up the hill each day, only to have it fall down again and have to start over the next day. They often feel like they are functioning on "automatic pilot" and wonder what happened to the gratification they once experienced in medicine.

Case Example

Dr. Damon, a 49-year-old pediatrician, was in a single-specialty group practice and was functioning in a way that caused increasing concern among his colleagues in the group. As far as they could tell, he continued to provide competent patient care, but they were worried about changes they noted in him. They sensed that he was simply "punching the time clock" and had lost any enthusiasm he once had for the practice of medicine. There was a grimness to him that was new and different. He seemed "cranky" in the office, and the office staff had to approach him cautiously because they sensed he was a bit more fragile than he had been before. He did not consult with his colleagues about difficult or challenging cases as he had in the past, and he did not seem to want to socialize with the other doctors in the group anymore. The office manager noted that he had not taken a vacation in a long time and was away from the office only if he were attending a continuing medical education meeting. He also seemed to be the first one in the office in the morning and the last one to leave in the evening. When two colleagues sat down with Dr. Damon for a cup of coffee, they shared their observations about him and expressed concern about him. He said he worked long hours because he could not get all the paperwork done in the time allotted for it, and he did not take vacations because he had no interest in going anywhere. They were candid in expressing their opinion that he was experiencing some kind of burnout or depression, and they talked him into seeing a psychiatrist for a consultation.

Dr. Damon made the appointment and saw a psychiatrist 2 weeks after the meeting with his colleagues. At first he said he was there only because his colleagues talked him into it, but after a few defensive opening remarks, he rapidly loosened up, and the psychiatrist felt that the floodgates had opened. He ventilated about his disillusionment with the practice of medicine. He linked it to a lawsuit that had occurred 2 years previously for what he described as a completely frivolous complaint. He expressed a sense that there was a grave injustice in the way that malpractice suits were handled in the United States. He said that no one had been more dedicated to his patients than he. He said he had been one of the top students in his medical school class and the best resident in his pediatrics program. He read all the journals and kept up to date like no one else. He said that it was completely unfair that the malpractice suit, which was ultimately dismissed, was listed in the National Practitioner Data Bank as a black mark against him.

He recalled the early days of medical school and residency, when he was highly idealistic and thought that if he did everything he was supposed to do, he would be appreciated and valued by patients and colleagues alike. He said that the family that sued him had taken three of their children to him over the years, and he had worked tirelessly to give them the best pediatric care available. The lawsuit struck him as "a slap in the face" and a sign of an extraordinary lack of gratitude. It made him convinced that he needed to work harder, and he expanded his hours, devoted himself diligently to the literature, and became obsessional in his documentation so that if he were ever sued again, he would be completely protected. The psychiatrist pointed out to him that the lawsuit appeared to confirm his longstanding sense of self-doubt—in other words, it proved that he was not as good as he should be. Dr. Damon acknowledged that he was highly perfectionistic and never felt that he measured up to his own expectations. He and the psychiatrist embarked on a course of psychotherapy in which Dr. Damon spent a good deal of time recounting the pressures he felt from his mother and father to be the perfect child to make up for serious problems in his brother. After 19 months of psychotherapy, Dr. Damon felt he had gained a great deal of insight and had much of his enthusiasm for medicine restored.

Midcareer burnout, as in Dr. Damon's case, is all too common and in many cases goes unnoticed and undiagnosed. Some physicians retire early from the practice of medicine or shift careers as a result of this burnout. Often they feel that the promise of reward has been retracted and that they were misled by their professors or role models early in their careers. Fortunately, psychotherapy appears to be effective when used in the treatment of OCPD. In a Scandinavian study using a randomized controlled design (Svartberg et al. 2004), 50 patients with Cluster C personality disorders were randomly assigned to 40 sessions of dynamic psychotherapy or cognitive therapy. Both treatments showed efficacy, and many of the patients were diagnosed with OCPD. Despite these encouraging findings, perfectionism is often difficult to treat and may require therapy that is extended beyond 40 sessions to modify the intensely held expectations of extraordinary performance. More of the details of the psychotherapy are discussed in Chapter 8 and Chapter 9 ("Individual Cognitive Therapy and Relapse Prevention Treatment").

No medications have been shown to be effective in OCPD, but when a clinically diagnosable major depressive disorder is present, an antidepressant may be useful. The syndrome of burnout may or may not be equivalent to clinical depression. There is overlap between burnout and depression, but they are not the same thing.

Sharing the Diagnosis With the Patient

The diagnosis of a personality disorder is rarely welcomed by the physician-patient. The term has pejorative connotations stemming from the tradition of using the term "character disorder" synonymously with "psychopath." Hence "personality disorder" often connotes moral turpitude or depravity rather than a complex syndrome stemming from genetic factors, early adverse experience, and struggles with self-development. Moreover, physician-patients are familiar with the diagnostic nomenclature, and through their rotations in psychiatry, they have experienced the pejorative implications of terms like "narcissistic" and "borderline."

A good strategy when sharing the diagnosis with the physician-patient is to approach the diagnostic understanding developmentally. It frequently helps, for example, to note how early adverse experiences shape a particular world view and lead to struggles with a secure sense of self. If the physician-patient understands that self-esteem grows out of a secure relationship with parents, it becomes understandable that a need for validation or affirmation persists. The various personality traits associated with the diagnosis can also be discussed in depth before applying any label. In many cases, there are features of more than one personality disorder, and the term "mixed personality disorder" can justifiably be applied. This term may be accepted more readily by physicians than either narcissistic personality disorder or BPD. However, if the diagnosis is clearly one or the other, the diagnosis can be shared after a detailed discussion of the psychological features of the condition. The evaluating clinician can openly acknowledge that pejorative connotations are sometimes associated with the diagnosis but can also clarify that they are unjustified prejudices—an example of the stigma associated with some psychiatric disorders. It may also help to explain to the physician-patient that the diagnosis of personality disorder does not automatically mean that a licensing board will see the physician as impaired. In any case, considerable time may need to be allotted to help the physician-patient work through the experience of being diagnosed with a personality disorder and process the reaction that it produces.

Key Points

- A variety of behaviors that involve lack of professionalism are commonly grouped under the term *disruptive physician*. Many of these behaviors reflect longstanding patterns associated with personality disorders or personality traits.

- Not all personality disorders manifest themselves in disruptive behaviors—some lead to patterns of burnout and depression.

- The insensitivity of narcissistic personality disorder often reflects an underlying insecurity, self-doubt, and inadequate self development.

- Narcissistic personality disorder and borderline personality disorder (BPD) both involve problems with mentalizing—that is, difficulties understanding how behaviors and comments affect others in the work setting.

- Although many narcissistic personality-disordered physicians are amenable to treatment, those with antisocial features are likely to be corrupt and not suitable for a career in medicine.
- Physicians with BPD are characterized by impulsivity, affective lability, chaotic relationships, and suicidality. Randomized controlled trials suggest that combinations of disorder-specific psychotherapy and selective serotonin reuptake inhibitors may be helpful.
- Obsessive-compulsive personality disorder, characterized by excessive perfectionism and rigidity, may lead to burnout and depression in mid-life.

Professional Boundary Violations

The concept of professional boundaries has been given increasing attention in recent decades. The Medical Board of California examined records of physicians disciplined from October 1995 to April 1997 (Morrison and Wickersham 1998), and 465 separate offenses were identified. The most common involved incompetence or negligence and abuse of alcohol or other drugs. However, professional boundary violations involving inappropriate prescribing practices (11%) and inappropriate contact with patients (10%) were in third and fourth place, respectively. In another survey of physicians disciplined for sex-related offenses (Dehlendorf and Wolfe 1998), it was noted that the number of physicians disciplined per year for sex-related offenses increased from 42 in 1989 to 147 in 1996. Moreover, the discipline handed out for sex-related offenses was much harsher than for non-sex-related offenses; 71.9% of sex-related sanctions involved revocation, surrender, or suspension of medical license.

These figures suggest that both sexual and nonsexual boundary violations are increasingly brought to the attention of licensing boards and are being taken seriously after a long era in which these kinds of transgressions largely flew under the radar. Indeed, many middle-aged physicians currently in practice received no training whatsoever in professional boundaries during medical school or residency training. Taking the Hippocratic oath certainly does not guarantee that one will refrain from professional misconduct, and the profession has now recognized the need to take preventive measures in training and

113

continuing education settings, to provide disciplinary responses to boundary violations in practice, and to design rehabilitation programs for those who are motivated to change.

Boundary violations have been the subject of a considerable number of contributions to the psychiatric literature for some time now (Epstein 1994; Epstein and Simon 1990; Frick 1994; Gabbard 1994; Gabbard and Lester 2003; Gutheil and Gabbard 1993). Professional boundaries as they apply to nonpsychiatric physicians have been more controversial, and the literature has only recently caught up to the comparable writings from psychiatry (Bloom et al. 1999; Gabbard and Martinez 2005; Gabbard and Nadelson 1995; Gartrell et al. 1992; Wilbers et al. 1992).

The term *boundaries* in medical practice are used in a variety of different ways. Although there is no totally consensual definition, a useful one developed by Gabbard and Nadelson (1995) is the following: "The parameters that describe the limits of a fiduciary relationship in which one person (a patient) entrusts his or her welfare to another (the physician) to whom a fee is paid for the provision of a service" (p.1445). Inherent in this definition is the acknowledgement of the power differential. This power imbalance is present even when one physician treats another. A physician is entrusted with the physical and mental health of a patient who is in a less powerful position by virtue of lacking the knowledge, experience, and professional training of the physician. The potential to exploit the patient's dependency is an ever-present risk. Hence the physician assumes an ethical position in which the patient's needs are placed before the physician's needs. Sexual involvement with patients is never considered ethical, given that it would constitute exploitation of the patient's trust. Moreover, informed consent is not possible because it may seem impossible to say no to someone who is treating you. Sexual exploitation is only the most extreme form of boundary violation. A variety of nonsexual boundary violations must be taken into account as well. These include dual relationships, business transactions, certain types of gifts and services, some forms of language use, some types of physical contact, the time and duration of appointments, the mishandling of fees, excessive self-disclosure, and the misuses of the physical examination (Gabbard and Nadelson 1995).

Most boundaries that attempt to outline the limits of the professional relationship cannot be rigidly applied in an unthinking way. It is important for physicians to be able to express their humanness in a variety of situations, even when the boundaries must bend a bit to accommodate such behavior. If a physician informs a patient of a cancer diagnosis, and the patient begins to sob, it may be entirely appropriate (and ethical) for the physician to place an arm around the patient's shoulder and offer comfort. Accepting small and inexpensive gifts may be perfectly acceptable in many situations and not in any way compromise the physician's objectivity. These *boundary crossings*, which are humane and responsive to occasional situations arising in medical practice, are neither exploitative nor harmful to the patient. They must be differentiated from egregious *boundary violations* that do exploit the patient's vulnerability and cause harm to the patient. The term *boundary transgressions* is sometimes used as an overarching concept that encompasses both variants. Minor boundary crossings occur regularly, and they must always be considered in context before leaping to the conclusion that a physician has made a serious boundary violation. Moreover, there can be boundary transgressions that involve honest misunderstandings, whereas others may be fueled by corrupt and unethical motives. These must be differentiated by carefully examining the context and the individuals involved.

The study of nonsexual boundary violations among physicians is essential for two reasons. Nonsexual boundary violations in and of themselves may cause harm to patients. Engaging in business transactions, for example, may permanently alter the physician–patient relationship in a way that leads to less-than-optimal care. Second, cases of sexual boundary violations by physicians who have been evaluated often reveal preexisting boundary violations of a nonsexual nature. This "slippery slope" phenomenon (Gabbard 1994; Gutheil and Gabbard 1993; Strasburger et al. 1992) is, in fact, the usual case. It is unusual for no boundary violations whatsoever to be present when sexual relations between doctor and patient have begun. A more common development is a steady progression that goes from excessive self-disclosure by the physician to meetings outside the office, followed by hugs, kisses, and an increasing degree of physical contact, until sexual relations are a regular occurrence. Thorough familiarity with nonsexual boundary violations may allow a physician to utilize them as early warning signals that he or she is becoming overinvolved with a patient *before* the relationship progresses to frank sexual misconduct (Gabbard and Nadelson 1995).

Sexual Boundary Violations

The American Medical Association (AMA) Council on Ethical and Judicial Affairs issued a 1991 statement: "Sexual contact or a romantic relationship concurrent with the physician–patient relationship is unethical" (American Medical Association Council on Ethical and Judicial Affairs 1991, p. 2741). In other words, no form of sexual contact between doctor and patient is acceptable under any circumstances. Such behavior interferes with the provision of good medical care to patients and exploits the dependency and the power differential inherent in the doctor–patient relationship.

A recent statement on sexual misconduct by the Federation of State Medical Boards outlines two broad types of professional sexual misconduct: sexual violation and sexual impropriety (Federation of State Medical Boards 2006). Both can be the cause of disciplinary action by a state medical board. *Sexual impropriety* involves making sexually demeaning comments to a patient, being disrespectful of the patient's privacy by not using appropriate disrobing or draping practices, using sexually suggestive expressions, or engaging in behavior that can be construed as sexual. Examples are such things as commenting on a patient's breasts in a sexualized way, examining the genital area without the use of gloves, or performing a breast or pelvic examination without clinical justification.

Sexual violation, on the other hand, is defined as something involving frank physical contact of a sexual nature between doctor and patient. It does not matter if the behavior is initiated by the patient or the doctor. In the federation guidelines, this behavior could include penetration, oral sex, or passionate, sexualized kissing.

One of the core principles in evaluating instances of sexual misconduct is that the feelings of doctor and patient, whatever they may be, are irrelevant to the determination of whether a boundary violation has occurred. In other words, even if a physician and a patient fall madly in love with each other, and both wish to engage in sexual relations, the sexual contact is still an unethical act. In fact, the AMA statement and the guidelines of the Federation of State Medical Boards cast a broad net. A rural primary care practitioner may be the only doctor in town, but if this physician dates a patient currently in treatment, the physician has committed a boundary violation. The guidelines also relate to unscrupulous physicians who might rape or fondle a patient under anesthesia, physicians who misuse the physical examination, predatory physicians who ask patients out for dates during the course of an office visit or an emergency department examination, and those who suggest that sexual contact with the physician might have therapeutic value (Gabbard and Nadelson 1995).

Some physicians and patients will argue that the relationship is entirely consensual. Patients who are sexually involved with their physician may claim that there is no power imbalance and that their dependency is not being exploited in any way. However, Johnson (1993) pointed out that any argument that mutual consent exists stands "in sharp contrast to the implied presumption of disproportionate professional control underlying the AMA's opinion on sexual misconduct." In addition, McCullough et al. (1996) proposed a virtues-based ethical argument apart from consent issues: in the context of the doctor–patient relationship the professional virtues of self-effacement and self-sacrifice obligate the physician to avoid acting on sexual feelings toward patients. Even if one could argue that in some cases the harm is not apparent, ethics codes are established based on a significant potential for harm, rather than on its certainty. By analogy, drunk driving laws are established because the majority of drivers are not able to safely steer an automobile from a bar to their home without having an accident.

Although some drivers may be able to drink a quart of hard liquor and drive from a tavern to their house without incident, the laws still make good sense.

Psychiatric Evaluation of Sexual Misconduct Cases

Most physicians charged with sexual misconduct come to psychiatric evaluation by way of a referral from a state board or, in Canada, a provincial college. In some cases, a physician's health program may handle a sexual misconduct complaint, but increasingly these transgressions are being seen as sufficiently serious that licensing boards must be involved. Other cases are referred from hospital risk management or medical staff committees. Still other cases, albeit a minority, involve a physician who realizes that an error in judgment has occurred and seeks help voluntarily to prevent any future occurrence of similar boundary violations. These physicians are filled with remorse and regret, and they recognize that they have behaved unethically. In a small number of states, the requirement to report mandated by state law may override considerations of doctor–patient confidentiality, but in most venues the evaluating clinician needs to make a judgment call regarding whether breaking confidentiality and reporting the physician is warranted. One is constantly weighing the risk to the public safety versus the commitment to confidentiality. Inherent in such a decision is an assessment of whether the physician is likely to repeat the behavior and whether he or she appreciates the harm done to patients. An alternative, of course, is to advise the physician to self-report.

A good starting point in determining whether the requirement to report sexual misconduct overrides doctor–patient confidentiality is to check state or provincial statutes. These vary widely. In Canada, for example, Ontario mandates reporting of physician–patient sexual misconduct for all 24 regulated health professions, trumping any ethics code regarding confidentiality (see Celenza 2007). A different statute holds in the state of Wisconsin; there, therapists are required to request permission to report from a patient who has been a sexual exploitation victim at the hands of a previous treater. Clinicians who decide to report without checking their regulatory statutes may think they are doing the right thing only to end up at high risk for a lawsuit based on breach of confidentiality. A useful Web site where one can check civil and criminal codes is www.advocateweb.org.

Mental health evaluators should not be in the position of determining whether an accusation against the physician is accurate or not. A clinician cannot be a detective or a judge. The investigation of the actual allegation can generally be conducted much more efficiently by state licensing boards or provincial colleges of physicians and surgeons. False accusations do exist, but they probably constitute a small number of the allegations made. No good data exist on the subject, but most patients will not go to the trouble of making a complaint if there is not some validity to it. In any case, the clinician conducting the evaluation is assessing the behavior in terms of motives and underlying psychopathology and evaluating whether the physician is likely to be a good candidate for a rehabilitation program. Evaluation should also take into account the risk of recurrence of such behavior.

Having stated that physicians who engage in sexual boundary violations do so for a variety of reasons, most physicians will fall into one of four categories: 1) psychotic disorders, 2) predatory psychopathy and paraphilias, 3) lovesickness, and 4) masochistic surrender (Gabbard and Lester 2003; see Table 7–1).

Psychotic Disorders

The psychotic disorders category is by far the rarest that one sees when evaluating physicians who have engaged in sex with patients. At times a manic episode with its associated hypersexuality may lead to poor judgment with a patient. Psychotic brain syndromes with frontal lobe involvement may also be responsible. However, these situations demand careful assessment, often with collaborative information or objective observations of others to make certain that the physician is not using his or her medical knowledge about symptoms of illness to rationalize unacceptable behavior.

Predatory Psychopathy and Paraphilias

Under the category "predatory psychopathy and paraphilias" we are not limiting ourselves to a narrow definition of psychopathy or true antisocial personality disorder. Rather, we are including sexual behavior that is psychopathic and predatory in nature, in that the physician is acting on sexual impulses without remorse for the harm done or empathy for the patient's experience of being exploited. These physicians, usually male, have often had a longstanding pattern of serially preying on others and discarding them when they lose interest. Hence severe narcissistic personality disorders with antisocial features would be included in this group as well. We include paraphilias not because we think that all those with paraphilias are psychopathic, but because those who enact their paraphilic urges *with patients* tend to have the same character structure involving lack of remorse and failure of empathy for the patient typical of the predator. A physician with a foot fetish, for example, who systematically finds false reasons to examine his patients' feet is acting in a predatory manner to gratify his own sexual desire.

Individuals in this category may have been identified in medical school or residency training as corrupt or dishonest in some way. They may have falsified medical records, lied to training directors about their whereabouts when they

---

TABLE 7–1. Categories of physicians who engage in sexual boundary violations

- Psychotic disorders
- Predatory psychopathy and paraphilias
- Lovesickness
- Masochistic surrender

---

missed call, or sold illegally acquired drugs to support their way through school. They may be masters at using threats of litigation to intimidate others when various transgressions are discovered. As a result, no one is willing to come forward as a complainant or witness.

Case Example

Dr. Phillips was a 46-year-old obstetrician-gynecologist who had complaints from four different patients that he had taken advantage of their vulnerability by starting up a sexual relationship with them. Each of them described similar behavior in the examination room. He would come into the room without a female chaperone present and talk very sympathetically to them about their concerns while stroking their hair with his fingers. He would tell them that they deserved more attention from their husbands and that they were "a real catch" or some similar phrase. Dr. Phillips would take an inordinately long time doing the pelvic exams, and some of the women described his putting his thumb on their clitoris during the actual examination as though he were attempting to stimulate them sexually. In each case he would ask the women if they would like to go for a drink after work, having scheduled them late in the afternoon and telling them that he was about to finish up his work for the day. The women were initially impressed by his charm and his seeming capacity to listen and care about their concerns. In each case, the drink after work led to a series of secret meetings in which he systematically seduced the women and then tried to end the relationship by explaining to the women that they could end his career if they would tell the licensing board about what he had done. He tried to enlist them in maintaining the secret so that he could continue his profession, making them feel responsible for his well-being. Several of the women felt that he was promising a more permanent relationship and felt betrayed by him. When one said she would file a complaint, he threatened to call her husband and claim that she had seduced him. When Dr. Phillips was evaluated, he denied the charges and indicated that the women had conspired against him with the idea of blackmailing him or suing him. He admitted to outside meetings with several of the women, but he insisted that they had initiated the meetings because they wanted to talk with him about their problems in greater detail than was possible in the office. His unconvincing lies were ultimately of no value when incriminating emails were discovered in the course of the investigation. Dr. Phillips then had his license revoked and has not returned to practice.

This example illustrates that in most cases involving this type of predatory behavior, there are multiple victims, and the physician is without remorse. Frequently, he will attempt to convince evaluators that he has actually been victimized, both by the state licensing board and by the patients. When patients inform the physician that they are going to complain, he may enlist an attorney to threaten them and indicate that they would be ruined if they file a complaint. They may be told that their entire sexual history will be revealed in an investigation by the state licensing board. These essentially corrupt and unethical physicians are not amenable to rehabilitation and are best counseled to look for other professions. In many states they will also face criminal charges for sexual battery.

Lovesickness

Physicians who fall in love with their patients are often in the throes of life crises. They may be going through a divorce, separation, a grief process in the face of a recent family member's death, or a serious illness in child or spouse. There may be serious financial setbacks, malpractice suits, or a sense of despair about their practice. Midlife disillusionment with medicine may in some cases lead the physician to seek escape by falling in love with a patient who seems to offer gratifications unavailable elsewhere.

As noted in Chapter 1 ("The Psychology of Physicians and the Culture of Medicine"), many "perfectionist" physicians seek an ill-defined reward for their selfless efforts at helping others. One middle-aged internist reflected on his transgression during the psychiatric evaluation. Filled with regret and remorse, knowing that what he did was unethical, he made the following observation: "All my life I have done my best to be there for my patients. I have sacrificed my own self-interest to help others. I have neglected my children and my wife to try to serve my patients. I found myself turning 50 and feeling that no one appreciates what I did for them. I felt like maybe I was entitled to one small self-indulgence, by actually thinking of myself first and acting on my feelings of love and passion for my patient."

When the physician is a female, a common pattern is for her to be charmed by a young man who is plagued with problems, such as addiction, personality disorder, and even legal trouble (Gabbard and Lester 2003). The female physician believes that he is simply a "baby" who needs the love of a good mothering figure. She may have a fantasy of settling him down and making him grow up. She may ultimately fall in love with this charming rogue and sacrifice her own career to rescue him from his difficulties. Indeed, the role of rescuer comes naturally to many physicians, and there is only a thin line between rescuing and sliding into feelings of love for a patient.

Other female physicians fall for a female patient, even though they consider themselves heterosexual. In the intensity of the doctor–patient relationship, they may feel that they have met their "soul mate" and seek a special bond with this patient, especially if there is a dead marriage at home with a man who appears to be uninterested. Most female physicians in this scenario do not initially think of themselves as "in love" or under the influence of erotic passion.

> Dr. Stanley was a 53-year-old family practitioner who lamented the fact that she did not have enough time for her patients, so she constantly stretched the sessions beyond what she should and ran late throughout her workday. Nevertheless, her patients felt she cared, and they would pour out their hearts to her with her encouragement. She typically did not arrive home in the evening until 8:00 or 8:30, and her husband had already eaten alone and would then spend his evenings on the computer. Hence she felt there was no companionship in her life, leaving her to spend more time at the office, where she felt there was some emotional connection with her patients. One patient, Georgia, became particularly attached to Dr. Stanley after her husband dumped her for another woman. She cried as she told Dr. Stanley about the circumstances. Georgia said to her: "You are the most comforting person in my life." She gave her doctor a hug at the end of her office appointment and told her she loved her. Without thinking, Dr. Stanley said, "I love you, too."
>
> Dr. Stanley encouraged Georgia to return so that they could talk further about what she was going through and monitor the antidepressant that Dr. Stanley had prescribed. In the next office visit, Georgia told Dr. Stanley how empty her life was, sitting in her house alone. Dr. Stanley was moved and told her that she herself had been divorced in her early 30s and had gone through similar pain. Georgia said that she had never felt so understood. Dr. Stanley then offered to get together with her over the weekend and do some shopping together since Georgia complained that she had no friends and was finding the weekends intolerable. They grew closer and sent each other E-mails daily in which they talked about mutual feelings of love and closeness—both felt that they were so much alike that they could read each other's minds. Dr. Stanley told Georgia that she knew what she was going to say before she even said it. They compared notes on their many similar interests and spent more and more time together outside the office. Intense hugs led to kisses and to caresses in the genital area, and both were frankly surprised at the erotic longing that emerged. As things deepened, Dr. Stanley explained to Georgia that it was not ethical to have a sexual relationship with a patient, and they needed to break it off before it progressed further. Georgia was enraged and felt betrayed by Dr. Stanley. She talked to her pastor about it, and he suggested that she contact the licensing board about Dr. Stanley.

The scenario in this case typifies the "slippery slope" pattern in the evolution of boundary violations of the lovesick type. Things begin with a preexisting vulnerability in the physician. Dr. Stanley had an empty marriage and found gratification in a patient who needed her. The rescue attempt led to excessive self-disclosure on her part, hugs, socializing outside the office, and passionate feelings of merger wherein they could actually read each other's minds. As things began to sexualize, she had the good sense to stop. However, the cessation trauma (Gutheil and Gabbard 1993) led Georgia to feel enraged and betrayed.

Masochistic Surrender

Although the physician is always responsible for maintaining professional boundaries, even when the patient is frankly seductive, many physicians feel they have been bullied or seduced into a relationship with a patient. They may protest to the licensing board that they had no alternative and that the patient would have committed suicide if they had not complied with his or her wishes. Certain physicians go to extraordinary lengths to help particularly difficult patients, only to feel tormented by the patient's demands (Gabbard and Lester 2003). These physicians are ordinarily troubled by any expression of their own aggression. As Karl Menninger (1957) once noted, the practice of medicine affords "a unique opportunity to conceal conscious or unconscious sadism" (p. 101). Workaholics often need to be loved by everyone (Rhoads 1977). When a demanding patient places extraordinary expectations on the doctor, the physician may feel obligated to appease the patient by meeting those demands.

Case Example

Dr. James was a 39-year-old psychiatrist who was treating a patient with borderline personality disorder in combined psychotherapy and pharmacotherapy. She became extremely angry at Dr. James when he ended the therapy hour right on time so that he could stick to his schedule. She told him that she felt like she was just another patient to him and that he was good at faking care and concern. He protested that even though he was paid for his work, he still felt real compassion for her. She responded that, "Even if you hated me, you would never show it. For all I know, I'm just seeing your professional role." He gradually extended the sessions by a few minutes to demonstrate to her that he actually cared about her and was not just functioning in a robotic manner that was part of a professional demeanor that he assumed at the office. She continued to demand more from him, including self-disclosures about his private life, which he assiduously avoided. The patient was divorced and insisted on knowing if Dr. James had been divorced. On one particular occasion she arrived at the office and stood in the middle of his waiting room, sobbing. He went to the waiting room and took her by the hand to lead her into the office. She said, "I have to have a hug." He responded by hugging her, knowing that he was probably making a mistake. She held on to him with a viselike grip and did not want to let him go. She explained that her cat had died, and she claimed that her cat was her only friend. She said that she felt her life was over and she might as well commit suicide. He sat on the couch in his office with her and held her while she sobbed. She said that she was convinced that suicide was the only option. He advised inpatient treatment, but she refused to go in the hospital. Dr. James let her leave the office only on the condition that she would call if she felt like she was going to act on her suicidal urges. That night she called him as he was preparing for bed, and she insisted that he come over to her apartment or she would end her life with an overdose of pills. He was filled with anxiety at the specter of a lawsuit from her family, and against his better judgment, he went to her apartment. While he was there, she clung to him and said that she needed to be held all night long. She let him know for the first time that she had been an incest victim and always regarded herself as "damaged goods." She said that no man would be interested in her because of that, and she saw her future as bleak and hopeless. He held her and finally said that he must leave. He offered to take her to the hospital. She said she would definitely kill herself if he left. Dr. James felt trapped. She unzipped his pants and performed fellatio on him. He found himself enjoying it, despite his intense anxiety that what he was doing was wrong and that he was going to get sued. She fell asleep at 3:00 A.M., and he gently left her apartment and went home. He called her in the morning and said that he could not continue to be her doctor because he had made a serious error in judgment. He referred her to a colleague. She said she was furious at him for "using me and throwing me away," and she filed a complaint against him with the licensing board.

Like the lovesick physician, those doctors who are involved in this scenario of progressively giving in to the demands of an aggressive and bullying patient usually only have a history of a transgression with one patient. They are not predators who have multiple victims in their practice. When Dr. James came to psychotherapy after an evaluation, he explored his difficulties with his own aggression. At one point, he recognized that he had tried to manage his anger by seeing it only in his patient and attempting to appease her to keep the rage from spilling over and destroying her as well as him. In this regard, she was being a container into which he could project all his own aggression.

This particular scenario also underscores the role that sexual abuse may play in the pathogenesis of boundary violations. Although we can never blame the patient for the transgression of a physician, those patients with a history of sexual victimization in childhood are at high risk for unconsciously reenacting their past in their relationship with the doctor (Gabbard and Lester 2003). For many incest victims, being cared about and sex are inextricably bound together. The patient may be overtly seductive or demanding in such a way that the doctor feels trapped into responding. The combination of the history of childhood sexual abuse and the doctor's difficulties in setting limits because of the feeling that they are too aggressive can be a fertile field for the development of sexual boundary violations. Victims of incest and child abuse have long been known to have a pattern of victimization, including sexual exploitation by therapists at higher rates (Browne and Finkelhor 1986; van der Kolk 1989). The internal world of a childhood sexual abuse victim is populated with three principal representations: abuser, victim, and rescuer (Gabbard 2005). These figures are internal self and object representations that are projected into the therapist and then re-introjected by the patient. The case involving Dr. James had him in the role of the patient's rescuer initially. However, as things progressed and her demands increased, she became identified with the internal abuser representation, and Dr. James began to feel victimized by her. Ultimately, Dr. James became the abuser when he reenacted the incestuous scenario from the past (Gabbard 2005b).

These four common categories of physicians who transgress sexual boundaries are not etched in granite. Some physicians will have characteristics of more than one category. Others seem to fall between the cracks of this classification and are not easily understood using these models. Any of these categories can also be found in conjunction with serious drug or alcohol abuse. Chemical substances may disinhibit a physician, leading to sexual behavior that would not have otherwise occurred. Hence part of a thorough evaluation of a sexual boundary violation is to carefully assess the role that substances may play in the scenario that unfolded.

Sexual Relations With Former Patients

Sexual relations between a physician and a current patient are always unethical. For psychiatric physicians, the American Psychiatric Association has declared, "Once a patient, always a patient"—in other words, there is an absolute ban on posttermination sexual relationships. The AMA Council on Ethical and Judicial Affairs makes it somewhat more ambiguous: "Sexual contact or a romantic relationship with a former patient may be unethical under certain circumstances" (American Medical Association Council on Ethical and Judicial Affairs 1991, p. 2741). This determination for nonpsychiatric physicians implies that individualized case review is necessary to ascertain whether there is exploitation of emotional dependency that continues in the physician–patient relationship. A one-time contact with an ophthalmologist or an emergency department physician may be of little emotional importance to many patients, so if the patient and the physician meet up years later, it would be hard to argue that exploitation is occurring. However, in other cases, the determination of exploitation is more complex. If, for example, a patient sees a surgeon for only one procedure but the patient's life is saved, there may be intense emotional feelings and persistent idealization long after the surgery (Gabbard and Nadelson 1995).

Many situations are ambiguous, however, and it may be difficult to determine whether misconduct has occurred from outside the relationship. Moreover, many patients will insist that there is no emotional dependency whatsoever and no power differential, as noted previously. Hence any physician who is contemplating a relationship with a patient must first terminate the doctor–patient relationship and allow a reasonable interval of time to pass. If a small-town primary care practitioner develops an interest in a patient, he or she may argue that there are no other doctors in town to treat the patient. However, if a romantic relationship is being considered, at the very least, the doctor should refer the patient to another physician in a neighboring town.

Most cases of posttermination sexual relations involve a doctor who ends the professional physician–patient relationship for the purpose of pursuing a sexual relationship. Many physicians who are intensely involved with a patient may terminate the doctor–patient relationship to avoid discipline from their licensing board. Often there are medical records or observations by office staff that convincingly demonstrate that a sexual romantic relationship was going on prior to the date of termination cited by the physician.

Assessment of Amenability to Rehabilitation

Sexual boundary violations are extraordinarily serious events in the practice of medicine. Yet it would be unfortunate if all physicians who engage in such violations were automatically considered unfit to practice, throwing away years of expensive education and training without a careful assessment. Those whose involvement is limited to one patient, such as the majority of the lovesick and masochistic surrender types, may be filled with remorse and deeply motivated to avoid all future transgressions. An independent psychiatric evaluation is essential in most cases to determine the contributing factors to the sexual misconduct, the risk of repeating similar transgressions, and the suitability for a rehabilitation program. Such evaluation should be conducted by someone who does not know the physician and is entirely independent in formulating a judgment. These evaluators should be chosen by the licensing board or physicians' health organization and not by the physician or that physician's attorney. If the physician denies any sexual involvement with the complaining patient, there is little point in pursuing an evaluation for amenability to rehabilitation. The physician will wonder, "rehabilitation for what?"

A comprehensive evaluation of the sort described in Chapter 3 ("Psychiatric Evaluation of Physicians") is necessary to gain an understanding of the accused physician. The category of lovesickness does not necessarily mean that the physician is open to a treatment program. Physicians who are intoxicated with their patient may feel that it is "true love" and that there is therefore nothing to be addressed by treatment or rehabilitation. It may take a decline of the "honeymoon phase" of the relationship and entry into a period of disillusionment before they recognize the ethical problem inherent in the relationship. Several aspects of the situation must be taken into account regarding whether the physician is suitable for a rehabilitation program—how many times the behavior has occurred, whether one or more patients were involved, how long the relationship lasted, whether the physician-patient has insight into what happened, whether the physician has empathy for the harm caused to the patient, and whether there is genuine regret or remorse. Collateral information from as many sources as possible must be considered, because frequently there is a "he said, she said" character to the situation. What the patient alleges and what the physician acknowledges may be quite different.

Most important of all is the physician's attitude about what happened. Does the physician take full responsibility for the conduct and demonstrate profound remorse and empathy? Remorse must be rigorously differentiated from narcissistic mortification (Celenza and Gabbard 2003). Genuine remorse involves a sense of horror at the rationalizations one employed and a deep concern about harm done to the patient. Narcissistic mortification is concerned only with damage to one's reputation or self-regard. In many cases of narcissistic mortification, the physician is mainly concerned that he or she has been caught and therefore disgraced. Also, is the physician curious about the behavior and deeply dedicated to avoiding it in the future?

Deciding on disciplinary measures is the province of the licensing board. The clinician doing the psychiatric evaluation is primarily interested in understanding the presence of psychiatric problems and the potential for there to be treatment for them, as well as the suitability for rehabilitation. If the licensing board decides not to revoke a license and the evaluating clinician believes that there is a potential for rehabilitation, a number of monitoring approaches can be used to assure public safety (see Table 7–2). These are outlined in the Federation of State Medical Boards' (2006) guidelines. They include such things as a requirement that chaperones are routinely in attendance during the physician's history-taking and examination of the patient, supervision of the physician by a colleague in the workplace, and practice limitations recommended by the evaluator. These limitations may include such things as restriction of patients by gender (e.g., only male patients in the case of a male heterosexual physician); no pelvic, rectal, or breast examinations; or, in the case of a psychiatrist, commitment not to treat patients with certain diagnoses involving childhood abuse. There also needs to be a rehabilitation coordinator who receives reports from the supervisor and those in the workplace. On-site review by board investigators or the physician health program may be useful in addition to the other practice limitations.

Psychotherapy and pharmacotherapy may be recommended as well. One critically important aspect of the psychiatric evaluation is to determine whether a suicide risk is present. Some physicians experience such massive loss of face when their sexual boundary violation is discovered that they become suicidal. Hence antidepressant medication or even hospitalization can be needed. In most cases, psychotherapy will be an essential part of the rehabilitation program, to help the physician understand his or her vulnerabilities and learn how to detect warning signs at the risk of repeating what happened before. Education in boundary violations and professional boundaries in general may also be recommended, by attendance either at the various programs around North America that are designed to teach boundaries or at continuing education conferences. To preserve confidentiality in the psychotherapy, it is probably best that the psychotherapist simply report whether the physician is attending the psycho-

---

TABLE 7–2. Approaches to rehabilitation of physicians with sexual boundary violations

---

- Required chaperone
- Supervision by colleague in the workplace
- Practice limitations
- Appointment of rehabilitation coordinator
- On-site review by board investigators or physician health program
- Psychotherapy
- Pharmacotherapy if indicated
- Education on professional boundaries

---

therapy and making productive use of the process rather than reveal the details of content. Physicians who know that the details of their psychotherapy will be revealed may conceal critically important aspects of their sexual fantasies or wishes from the therapist. Psychotherapy of physicians who have engaged in sexual misconduct presents a host of challenges that are discussed in Chapter 8.

Nonsexual Boundary Violations

Most of the attention from regulatory bodies is focused on sexual boundary violations. In one study of 100 cases of professional boundary violations identified in physicians undergoing outpatient psychiatric evaluation (Gabbard and Martinez 2005), the investigators noted that 53 of the physicians had engaged in sexual boundary violations with patients. Nevertheless, there were a variety of other nonsexual violations that had caused major concern to patients, colleagues, office employees, hospital risk management committees, and other third parties. These included, for example, financial dealings with patients, social relationships, transgressions of confidentiality, and prescribing-related irregularities. As noted earlier, nonsexual boundary violations can be damaging in and of themselves as well as leading down the slippery slope to sexual misconduct. Here we consider some of the boundary issues that are relevant to these nonsexual categories.

Dual Relationships

Any kind of dual relationship has potential for damaging the doctor–patient alliance. However, just because the physician sees the patient in another context does not automatically indicate the presence of a boundary violation. The fundamental role of the physician is to make the patient's needs the first priority. The risk with dual relationships is that other needs may get in the way or interfere with the physician's objectivity. For this reason it is never a good idea for physicians to treat their own family members except in extreme emergencies. Similarly, physicians who accept the offer of a business relationship with a patient may contaminate their medical judgment when embarking on a partnership or investment program. For example, one physician who invested with his patient and lost a substantial sum of money ended up feeling deeply resentful that he had trusted this patient based on a good doctor–patient relationship. Both the friendship and the professional relationship were damaged, and ultimately the patient went elsewhere for medical care.

Some dual relationships may seem benign initially but can lead to unforeseen consequences. An academic physician may make a helpful gesture in treating a resident, but if she also must evaluate the resident's academic performance, problems may arise. A physician who prescribes for employees without having a doctor–patient relationship or a medical record may feel that she is doing a favor for the friend or employee. However, the friend or employee may feel that she is getting second-class medical care because there is no full history or physical examination preceding the decision to prescribe. Many licensing boards will discipline doctors who are treating people without a medical record. Moreover, because of the power differential, some patients may feel unable to say no to an offer from a doctor to have a social relationship. Patients may also misconstrue the doctor's intent. A physician who went to have coffee with the patient was seen as making a romantic overture to the patient when that was the farthest thing from his mind (Gabbard and Martinez 2005).

Dual relationships vary considerably from one culture to another. In certain countries outside North America, it is expected and commonplace that a doctor will have social relationships with patients, and there may be the culture shock associated with the different set of expectations in the United States or Canada. Educational curricula to familiarize international graduates with customs and expectations when they emigrate to North America may be extremely helpful in this regard (Myers 2004).

Time and Duration of Appointments

Professionalism includes consideration of the patient's schedule as well as the physician's. Maintaining an orderly schedule of patients' appointments and being punctual are reasonable expectations. The time and duration of appointments become problematic from the standpoint of boundaries when a particular patient is seen for a period of time that greatly exceeds the number of minutes allotted for the appointment. Another boundary issue can be the scheduling of the appointment late in the evening when office staff have gone home (Dr. Phillips is an example). Attorneys have noted that in many cases of sexual misconduct, the patient has been scheduled for the last appointment of the day when no one else is around. Such scheduling may be reflective of the potential for boundary violations (Gutheil and Gabbard 1993).

Excessive Self-Disclosure

Physicians often establish rapport by "chit-chatting" with their patients about matters of mutual interest. Some self-disclosure is warranted because it puts the patient at ease and helps establish a strong therapeutic alliance with the doctor. However, as illustrated in the foregoing cases of sexual boundary violations, when physicians talk about their personal problems with the patient, a role reversal is created in which the patient may feel ill at ease in trying to take care of the physician. Above all, the physician should not burden the patient. Hence physicians should be mindful of not using the patient as a sounding board to discuss their own problems. Another variation is the narcissistically oblivious physician who rambles on about his or her own life while ignoring the patient's need to be heard and understood.

Gifts and Donations

Physicians who solicit donations from patients place the patient in an awkward situation. Patients may well fear that they will not get good care unless they do as their doctor asks. If they *do* make a donation, they may feel entitled to special treatment. Physicians should abstain from active fundraising or other financial activities that make the patient feel obligated.

Many grateful patients wish to provide their physician with a small gift, and accepting such a gift graciously may be the best thing for the doctor–patient relationship. However, when large or expensive gifts are offered to the physician, or any amount of money, the physician needs to be wary. The gift-giving may involve a conscious or unconscious bribe designed to keep unpleasant subjects and negative feelings out of the doctor–patient relationship (Gabbard and Nadelson 1995). The physician's clinical judgment may be influenced by a large gift in the same way that gifts from pharmaceutical companies have been shown to influence physicians (Chren et al. 1989; Wazana and Primeau 2002).

Language

The use of certain kinds of language can feel like a boundary transgression to a patient. Some doctors use pet names or demeaning names such as "honey" or "sugar." There is already a loss of dignity when a patient assumes the patient role and has to disrobe and wear a gown in front of the doctor. Addressing patients with these types of diminutives may be experienced as a further loss of dignity (Gabbard and Nadelson 1995). Moreover, use of slang for genitals or breasts may be heard as seductive or offensive to some patients.

Physical Contact Other Than the Physical Examination

Shaking hands with a patient before or after the session is an entirely acceptable practice that rarely creates problems for the patient. However, hugs or kisses can become problematic. Physicians who hug their patients may raise false hopes in the minds of their patients about the intent of the physician for a different kind of relationship. Patients with a history of sexual abuse may be hypersensitive to any type of violation of boundaries. A hug or a kiss may even feel like an assault to them. Many physicians do not know if the patient in their examination room has been a childhood sexual abuse victim, and clear boundaries about physical contact besides the physical examination are prudent.

As noted earlier, certain situations in which a patient is deeply distressed may warrant a hand on the shoulder or a brief hug with the patient who initiates the hug. However, one cannot know in advance what the effect of a hug will be on the patient. One rule of thumb is not to initiate a hug but to accept a hug from the patient only after the patient initiates it and if the situation warrants it. Hugging should not be seen as a regular part of the doctor's visit either, because there may be an expectation of further contact as a result.

The Physical Examination

As we noted in the section on "Sexual Boundary Violations," sometimes the misuse of a physical examination can itself be regarded as a sexual boundary violation. The patient who presents with a sore throat and is given a breast examination may quite appropriately feel violated by the physician. The presence of a chaperone is a wise procedure in all physical examinations. Traditionally within medicine, a female chaperone is present when a male physician is examining a female patient. However, this advice is probably too general and does not allow for problems that arise in other gender constellations. There are several situations where it is good judgment to have a chaperone present: 1) with the patient who has a known history of sexual abuse, 2) with a patient undergoing a pelvic examination, 3) with a patient who is litigious, 4) with a patient who has considerable anxiety or a serious psychiatric illness, and 5) with a patient who for any reason raises concerns in the mind of the physician.

If there is a longstanding, solid relationship between doctor and patient, some of these considerations may not apply. Draping the patient appropriately for the physical examination is also essential. Finally, physicians must carefully explain the reason for examining the breasts, the genital area, or any other body part so the patient feels informed about the purpose of the particular procedure.

Evaluation of Nonsexual Boundary Violations

Complaints are less likely to be made about nonsexual boundary violations, although they appear to be more common now than in the past. In many geographical areas there are benign overprescribers who basically write a prescription for whatever the patient feels is necessary. Some of these physicians have difficulty with their aggression and are unable to say no to their patients. A different subgroup of physicians who overprescribe are essentially corrupt in trying to make money by "dealing drugs" to patients. These two different motives should be sorted out in the course of an evaluation. Also, education is needed about appropriate boundaries in prescribing and the need for a person who receives a prescription to be registered as a patient with a medical record. Clinicians who undertake mental health evaluations for doctors who have engaged in nonsexual boundary violations must assess whether education or treatment is the optimal approach. In light of the fact that professional boundaries have been taught in medical school and residency training only in the past couple of decades, many middle-aged and elderly physicians have had no education about boundaries. Many of them insist that they are simply doing what their role models did when they write prescriptions for colleagues in the corridors of the hospital or for employees who have a headache or other minor problem. Some physicians feel they are too busy to get to a doctor's office, so they treat themselves.

A frequent underlying issue in pervasive nonsexual boundary violations is a wish to be all things to all people. As noted in Chapter 1, physicians may have a secret omnipotence in which they feel they can meet the needs of everyone and gain the approbation and idealization they are longing for through meeting all the patient's demands. They may actually give money to patients who are broke or even have a patient stay in their house when the patient is homeless (Gabbard and Martinez 2005). Helping physicians accept limits and modify their omnipotence may require psychotherapy. Similarly, practice limitations often are needed as well as education through the monitoring of a physician's health program or licensing board to ensure that appropriate boundaries are implemented in the office. Direct on-site supervision from a senior colleague may be helpful as well. It is commonplace for both sexual and nonsexual boundary violations to be treated in part by discouragement of any kind of solo practice. Physicians who consistently violate boundaries will generally do much better in a group or institutional setting where there are role models and mentors available to them.

Key Points

- Sexual relations between a physician and a current patient are always unethical.

- Sexual relations between a physician and a patient after the ending of the doctor–patient relationship may be unethical and must be assessed on a case-by-case basis. In psychiatry, however, a sexual relationship with a former patient is always unethical.

- Many sexual boundary violations begin with the "slippery slope" of nonsexual boundary violations.

- Sexual misconduct cases should be sent for an independent psychiatric evaluation by someone who does not know the physician.

- Physicians who violate sexual boundaries tend to fall into one of four categories: psychotic disorders, predatory psychopathy and paraphilias, lovesickness, or masochistic surrender. Many physicians in the latter two categories are amenable to rehabilitation. Alcohol or drug abuse may disinhibit and contribute to sexual misconduct.

- Part of the psychiatric evaluation must assess the amenability to rehabilitation, and genuine remorse must be differentiated from narcissistic mortification.

- A psychiatric evaluation cannot decide the facts of what happened or determine disciplinary measures.

- Evaluation of nonsexual boundary violations should proceed in a similar manner to sexual boundary violations.

PART III

PREVENTION, GENERAL TREATMENT PRINCIPLES, AND REHABILITATION

Psychodynamic Psychotherapy

Psychodynamic psychotherapy is a time-honored treatment approach that derives from psychoanalysis and psychoanalytic technique. It is highly useful in the treatment of many physicians, but in this chapter we can offer little more than an introduction to the treatment itself. The reader is referred to a number of useful texts for further information (Book 1998; Gabbard 2004; Luborsky 1984; McWilliams 2004).

Psychodynamic psychotherapy is usually subdivided into two forms based on the duration of the treatment. Short-term psychodynamic psychotherapy (STPP) is generally regarded as a treatment that lasts 6 months or less, whereas long-term psychodynamic psychotherapy (LTPP) is a modality that has a longer duration and is often open-ended (Gabbard 2004). Regardless of length, psychodynamic psychotherapy is based on a set of principles that derive from psychoanalytic thinking (see Table 8–1).

General Principles

Much of Mental Life Is Unconscious

In most cases, when physicians are asked why they behave the way they do, their answer is simple: "I don't know." Much of what determines one's feelings, thoughts, and behaviors is beyond conscious awareness. Psychodynamic psychotherapy recognizes that patients are often consciously confused and unconsciously controlled (Gabbard 2005b).

Childhood Experiences Help Shape the Adult

All psychodynamic theories operate from a developmental premise—namely, that experiences in childhood are influential in determining who one is. There are a variety of different theoretical models with different perspectives on development. Regardless of one's preferred theory, however, one must take into account that genetic factors interact with early environmental influences to shape personality. A growing body of research (Caspi et al. 2002; Gabbard 2005a; Feinberg et al. 2007; Reiss et al. 1995) suggests that genes may be shut down or activated by environmental factors early in life. Other constructs, such as secure and insecure attachment, which is based on the mother or caregiver's own attachment classification, may also have far-reaching impact on the personality of the individual.

Transference Is a Primary Source of Understanding

One of the core principles of psychodynamic therapy is the construct of transference. Patients in treatment tend to attribute qualities associated with a figure from the past to the therapist. As a result, feelings about that figure are experienced in the same way with the therapist. Hence the therapeutic relationship provides an in vivo glimpse of the patient's characteristic patterns of relationships, and the focus on what transpires between patient and therapist may illuminate what goes on in other relationships outside the therapy.

Countertransference Provides Valuable Understanding About What Patient Induces in Others

The therapist's countertransference is similar to the patient's transference. The therapist unconsciously experiences a patient according to internal templates of figures from the therapist's past. Over time, the concept of countertransference has been expanded to include the therapist's reaction to the patient that is induced by the patient's behavior as well (Gabbard 1995a). Patients may behave in obnoxious or provocative ways that make the therapist angry, and the therapist's reaction says more about the patient's behavior than the therapist's actual past. In contemporary thinking, however, countertransference is usually seen as jointly created by what is induced in the therapist by the patient and the past figures in the therapist's life that continue to haunt the therapist as internal object representations.

TABLE 8–1.   Basic principles of psychodynamic psychotherapy

- Much of mental life is unconscious.

- Childhood experiences in concert with genetic factors shape the adult.

- The patient's transference to the therapist is a primary source of understanding.

- The therapist's countertransference provides valuable understanding about what the patient induces in others.

- The patient's resistance to the therapy process is a major focus of the therapy.

- Symptoms and behaviors serve multiple functions and are determined by complex and often unconscious forces.

- A psychodynamic therapist assists the patient in achieving a sense of authenticity and uniqueness.

Source.   Reprinted from Gabbard GO: *Long-Term Psychodynamic Psychotherapy: A Basic Text.* Washington, DC, American Psychiatric Publishing, 2004. Copyright 2004, American Psychiatric Publishing. Used with permission.

Resistance to the Therapy Process Is a Major Focus of Therapy

A fundamental aspect of psychodynamic therapy is the acknowledgement that patients are ambivalent about changing and therefore may resist the therapist's efforts to help. Patients have developed a set of defense mechanisms that protect them from intrapsychic pain, and when the patient is exposed to insight from the therapist, this new understanding may be highly threatening. Hence the patient may oppose the therapist's efforts to offer new perspectives on the patient's internal world. Defense mechanisms may become resistances when the patient enters psychotherapy. For example, a physician-patient who has developed obsessive-compulsive defenses, such as intellectualization and isolation of affect, may approach the psychotherapy in the same way. When the psychotherapist tries to help the physician get in touch with difficult feelings, the physician-patient may intellectualize and isolate any emotional states in such a way that the insight of the therapist is avoided.

Symptoms and Behaviors Serve Multiple Functions and Are Determined by Complex and Often Unconscious Forces

Psychodynamic psychotherapy is anti-reductionistic. In other words, the dynamic therapist recognizes that most symptoms and behaviors serve a number of functions and have a variety of causes and meanings that interact with one

another. Hence psychodynamic therapists are skeptical about accepting phenomena at face value without exploring the multiple contributions to whatever
the phenomena may appear to be.

The Psychodynamic Psychotherapist Assists the Patient in Achieving Authenticity and Uniqueness

Whereas descriptive psychiatry emphasizes how a number of symptoms form a
cluster typical of a syndrome that is shared by many patients, psychodynamic
psychiatry emphasizes how each individual is unique. Psychodynamic therapists help the patient develop a solid sense of self, however idiosyncratic and
different from others it may be. A search for authenticity and the multifaceted
nature of one's identity is instrumental to psychodynamic psychotherapy (Gabbard 2004).

When these factors are taken together, an in-depth approach to the human
psyche emerges. A useful definition that incorporates some of these basic elements is the following: "A therapy that involves careful attention to the therapist–patient interaction, with thoughtfully timed interpretation of transference
and resistance embedded in a sophisticated appreciation of the therapist's contribution to the two-person field" (Gunderson and Gabbard 1999, p. 685). Although interpretation is considered a key intervention in psychodynamic therapy,
it is not the only type of comment made by the therapist. A sensitive psychodynamic therapist varies the frequency and intensity of interpretation based on
the patient's capacity for insight. Indeed, psychodynamic therapy is often referred to as expressive-supportive therapy, and one can conceptualize a continuum of interventions that are used from the most interpretive or expressive to
the most supportive (see Figure 8–1).

Interpretation, at the expressive end of the continuum, attempts to make
conscious what has long been unconscious. Hence the therapist provides insight
into phenomena of behavior, thought, or feeling that were previously outside
the patient's conscious awareness. On the supportive end of the continuum, patients may require much more support and need advice and praise. In a typical
psychodynamic psychotherapy, the therapist shifts flexibly along this continuum based on the patient's capacities and the therapist's sense of timing.

Efficacy and Indications

The evidence base for psychodynamic psychotherapy is not as extensive as the
empirical support for cognitive-behavioral therapy (see Chapter 9, "Individual
Cognitive Therapy and Relapse Prevention Treatment"). Nevertheless, in recent

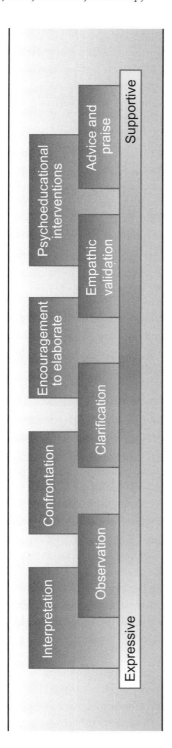

FIGURE 8–1. An expressive-supportive continuum of interventions.

Source. Reprinted from Gabbard GO: *Long-Term Psychodynamic Psychotherapy: A Basic Text.* Washington, DC, American Psychiatric Publishing, 2004, p. 63. Used with permission.

years a series of randomized, controlled trials have shown that STPP is efficacious in a number of specific disorders, including major depression, social phobia, panic disorder, generalized anxiety disorder, posttraumatic stress disorder, somatoform disorders, and bulimia nervosa (Leichsenring et al. 2004).

LTPP has a smaller evidence base because the length of the treatment creates formidable obstacles for conducting randomized, controlled trials, including the identification of a suitable control group, the cost of the study, and the problem of dropouts (Gunderson and Gabbard 1999). In spite of the difficulties, however, randomized, controlled trials support the use of LTPP in conditions such as borderline personality disorder and Cluster C personality disorders, which includes obsessive-compulsive, avoidant, and dependent personality disorders (Bateman and Fonagy 1999, 2001; Clarkin et al. 2007; Svartberg et al. 2004). Obsessive-compulsive personality disorder should not be confused with obsessive-compulsive disorder, which does not respond well to dynamic therapy. There are also randomized, controlled trials supporting the use of psychodynamic psychotherapy in conjunction with drug counseling in the treatment of substance-related disorders (Crits-Christoph et al. 2001).

Studies of LTPP, although few in number, suggest that improvements continue to accrue after termination. Follow-up data show that the therapist–patient dialogue appears to be internalized and results in continued changes in the patient 12–18 months later (Bateman and Fonagy 2001; Svartberg et al. 2004).

In psychodynamic psychotherapy, indications are not based simply on efficacy data. Psychodynamic assessment involves an evaluation of the personality of the physician to determine whether psychodynamic therapy is suitable. If the patients are not interested in some form of in-depth understanding, dynamic therapy may also be contraindicated. Some of the patient characteristics that augur well for a positive response to interpretive psychodynamic therapy include psychological mindedness, reasonably good judgment, the capacity to form meaningful relationships, an ability to use metaphor, reasonably good impulse control, and above-average intelligence (Gabbard 2005b). Even if a physician-patient possesses all these characteristics, an interpretive dynamic therapy may not be indicated if he or she comes to treatment in a state of crisis involving such stressors as a marital break-up, loss of a spouse, or a suspension of one's medical license. Therapists may need to use supportive interventions to shore up adaptive defense mechanisms and help the physician-patient successfully survive the current crisis. When the dust settles, the therapist may shift in some cases to a more expressive or interpretive emphasis.

Psychodynamic psychotherapy generally requires some degree of therapeutic alliance, that is, a willingness in the patient to ally him- or herself with the therapist in pursuit of common goals, and a perception by the patient of being helped. Extensive research (Hilsenroth 2007; Horvath 2005) has documented that the therapeutic alliance is one of the most potent predictors of outcome. Patients' assessments of the alliance (i.e., being helped by the therapist) tend to be more predictive of outcome than other sources. In fact, an early positive alliance is probably a better predictor than later measurements. Patients who are essentially forced into psychotherapy as part of an overall rehabilitation plan may have no sense of alliance and thus may not respond well. Therapists may feel discouraged under such circumstances. If there is at least a willingness to acknowledge that psychotherapeutic exploration may be productive and that one's own difficulties can be better understood, an extended trial of psychodynamic psychotherapy may be worth attempting. Even though data from randomized, controlled trials are lacking, clinical wisdom suggests that entrenched characterological features, such as those found in narcissistic and histrionic personality disorders as well as some mixed personality disorders, may be effectively treated with long-term psychodynamic strategies (Gabbard 2005b; Leichsenring, in press). Psychodynamic psychotherapy in physicians who have these entrenched features is generally offered as one component in a comprehensive rehabilitation and treatment plan so that other interventions are brought to bear in addition to the once- or twice-weekly therapy provided by the dynamic therapist.

Case Examples

Some clinical illustrations demonstrate the principles of psychodynamic therapy applied to instances of troubled physicians.

Dr. Damon

As the reader will recall from Chapter 6 ("Personality Disorders, Personality Traits, and Disruptive Physicians"), Dr. Damon was a 49-year-old pediatrician who was being sued after years of perfectionistic and meticulous work. His colleagues recognized signs of burnout occurring in Dr. Damon and suggested that he seek psychiatric consultation. Unlike many physicians, he dropped his defenses rather rapidly and readily formed a therapeutic alliance with Dr. Benjamin, his therapist, to examine his longstanding obsessive-compulsive personality features. Dr. Damon had suffered a deep wound to his self-esteem when a family sued him after he had selflessly taken care of their three children over the years and had viewed himself as a close friend of the family.

Even though Dr. Damon was motivated to understand himself, he began the therapy with his characteristic defenses operating as resistances. He led off with detailed accounts of the lawsuit and the case law associated with similar suits. His focus was on facts rather than feelings, and his efforts to be comprehensive often filled the entire 50-minute hour so that his therapist could not get a word in edgewise. Dr. Benjamin noted some irritation in himself. As he reflected on his countertransference, he realized that he felt completely controlled. He used his feelings to inform an observation he then made to Dr. Damon: "It feels like your need to tell me all the facts keeps you from painful feelings and keeps me from saying much of anything." Dr. Damon paused for a moment and acknowledged that he was anxious about what Dr. Benjamin might say or think.

Dr. Damon then said that he was deeply concerned that his colleagues had lost respect for him. Dr. Benjamin asked him what they had said to indicate their loss of respect. Dr. Damon replied that they had said nothing. On the contrary, his colleagues in his group repeatedly told him how much confidence they had in him. They viewed him as one of the best physicians in the community. The therapist then offered an interpretation that attempted to make what was unconscious more conscious: "I wonder, then, if the loss of respect you think you perceive in others is really your own loss of respect for yourself. After all, you failed at being perfect." Here Dr. Benjamin interpreted the defense mechanism of projection; by commenting that his patient "failed at being perfect," he was also helping Dr. Damon see the absurdity of striving for perfection.

Dr. Damon teared up with this insight and acknowledged that he was riddled with self-doubt. He had dealt with that self-doubt throughout his life by trying to be the best at what he did. He had a career trajectory in mind throughout his years of pediatric practice, and the lawsuit had totally shattered his view of where he should be. Dr. Benjamin noted that his patient had written something of a life script for himself long ago. This script amounted to an unconscious contract that if he devoted himself tirelessly to his patients, he would be loved and appreciated for it. Dr. Benjamin offered a bit of humor to soften the superego pressures: "You know what they say—if you want to make God laugh, tell Him your plans." Dr. Damon was able to chuckle through his tear-filled eyes.

After some time in therapy, Dr. Damon confided a transference fantasy to Dr. Benjamin. He worried that his therapist also viewed him as a failure, and he found himself expecting criticism from him when he came to the session. His therapist asked him if that fear reminded him of anything from his past. Dr. Damon responded that when he came home with his report card as a child, he always dreaded his father's reaction to his grades. If he had only one B in the context of a large number of As, his father would typically inquire as to what had happened in that one course that led to the B. Even though his father was not harshly or excessively critical, Dr. Damon experienced him as having been deeply disappointed.

Dr. Benjamin asked his patient if he felt that his demeanor in the therapy suggested that he was disappointed in Dr. Damon. After a few moments' reflection, Dr. Damon indicated that in fact, he felt accepted and supported by his therapist. He was frankly puzzled at the conviction that his therapist was viewing him as a failure. The therapist offered a transference interpretation: "I think what's happening here is typical of your life story; you attribute your own high expectation to everyone around you and then end up feeling tormented by not living up to what you imagine others expect of you."

Dr. Damon was more in touch with his feelings than many people with obsessive-compulsive personality traits. Perhaps because he was deep into self-examination as a result of a lawsuit, his affect states were less defended and more accessible. Nevertheless, Dr. Benjamin had to call his attention to the way his defenses were operating as resistances. His therapist also made good use of his countertransference feelings to alert him to the resistance. Dr. Benjamin was also systematically pointing out Dr. Damon's perfectionistic fantasies and his super-ego pressures. He used humor to help Dr. Damon take some distance from his high expectations, and he repeatedly pointed out how Dr. Damon's own self-doubt and excessive expectations of himself were projected onto others. An overriding strategy was to help Dr. Damon accept his humanness and limitations as well as the feelings he had that were unacceptable to him. Like many obsessive physicians, he used reaction formation as a way of defending against his own anger and aggression. He took care of children as a way of denying that he had any destructiveness within him. Through the psychotherapy, Dr. Damon discovered that the reason a malpractice suit was so devastating was that he feared that his own destructiveness, which he had so carefully defended against for years, was now obvious to everyone to see.

This case nicely fits a dynamic therapy model known as the "Core Conflictual Relationship Theme" (Book 1998; Luborsky 1984). The therapist looks for patterns of relationships in the patient's narratives. These often are organized along three components: a wish, a response from the other, and a response from the self. In Dr. Damon the wish was to please others by being perfect. The feared response from the other was disapproval. The response of the self was to work even harder and even more selflessly.

Dr. Sims

A frequent source of difficulties in disruptive physicians, particularly those with narcissistic and borderline personality traits, is problems with mentalization. As described in Chapter 6, such physicians are fundamentally clueless about the way they come across to others. They go through the workday oblivious to the impact they are having on those with whom they work, and often they are extraordinarily surprised to learn that complaints have been filed against them.

> Dr. Sims, the general surgeon described in Chapter 6, was prototypical of an incapacity to mentalize, and Dr. Jennings, the psychiatrist who evaluated him, did not initially think that Dr. Sims was likely to be suitable for psychodynamic therapy. However, after working with him in the evaluation, Dr. Jennings saw that there was a chink in Dr. Sims's defensive armor, an opening that allowed him to be reached. The surgeon was aware that he was increasingly becoming "irrelevant," because younger surgeons were challenging his preeminence in the hospital and women were not responding to him as they once had. Dr. Jennings outlined a treatment plan that was described in Chapter 6. One component was long-term dynamic psychotherapy that would increase his capacity to mentalize and expand his ability to engage in self-reflection.
>
> Dr. Sims began once-weekly sessions with Dr. Jennings, who forged a good therapeutic alliance by affirming that Dr. Sims was clearly a competent surgeon.

He also empathized with the feelings of limits accompanying the aging process. He allowed Dr. Sims to ventilate but challenged his point of view. When Dr. Sims spoke dogmatically in absolutist terms, Dr. Jennings would make comments like, "I imagine that others might see the situation somewhat differently." He thus demonstrated a mentalizing stance while modeling a willingness to understand in depth how Dr. Sims felt about himself. Dr. Jennings also expressed curiosity about the recent complaints brought against him. When Dr. Sims demeaned nurses and medical students for breaking down in tears when he confronted them, Dr. Jennings would ask, "What do you suppose is going on in their minds that led them to cry?"

Dr. Sims would respond with denigrating comments such as, "They're just pussies. They can't stand up to the criticism that they need to hear."

Dr. Jennings did not let it stay at that level of discourse. He continued to promote a mentalizing process in Dr. Sims. He asked, "You know, if they see you as a powerful and confident surgeon whose opinion they value, isn't it possible that they feel humiliated and intimidated by you?"

Dr. Sims bristled at this suggestion, and said, "I don't give a damn what they think—I'm just trying to make them better at what they do."

Dr. Jennings tried to open up a greater capacity for reflectiveness by pointing out, "Sometimes I don't think you pause and think about how you're coming across and how others experience you. I think there might be some shift in the way you're regarded and in the complaints that are filed about you if you considered how others perceive you differently than you perceive yourself." Dr. Sims responded, with some curiosity, "What do you mean exactly?" Dr. Jennings replied, "Well, I've noticed that sometimes you come across as though you're dismissing the validity of what I say, and I imagine that others might experience you similarly." Dr. Sims clarified that, in fact, he was not being dismissive and wanted to know what Dr. Jennings thought.

Dr. Jennings responded, "I'm glad to hear that you're interested in my perspective. It's an example of how I perceive you differently than how you generally perceive yourself."

In this brief vignette from the therapy, Dr. Jennings is using a technique known as "mentalizing the transference" (Bateman and Fonagy 2006). Dr. Jennings, in essence, was encouraging Dr. Sims to be curious about what is happening in the relationship in the present moment, specifically in terms of contrasting perspectives on his behavior. He used the transference relationship as an example of what happens in the hospital with Dr. Sims's colleagues and fellow employees. The emphasis was not on explaining how Dr. Sims came to feel as he does, but rather on expanding his thinking to include the subjectivity of his own and others' perceptions. Moreover, Dr. Jennings pointed out to him the practical advantages of taking into account how others saw him—namely, that it might decrease his level of complaints in the work setting. In addition to this mentalizing approach, he also helped Dr. Sims to mourn his lost youth and face the developmental tasks of middle age. He encouraged him to derive pleasure from mentoring others and to gain gratification from their success rather than focusing exclusively on his own achievements.

Dr. Stanley

Long-term psychodynamic psychotherapy is often the most useful and helpful treatment for physicians who have become involved in a sexual boundary violation, particularly when only one violation has occurred and the physician falls into the category of lovesickness or masochistic surrender. Dr. Stanley, described in Chapter 7 ("Professional Boundary Violations"), became involved with a needy female patient, whom she felt was her soul mate. In her pursuit of being a dedicated physician who ministered to the needs of her patients, she neglected her husband, who gradually disengaged from her and lived a life of solitude at the computer.

> After her transgression with Georgia, Dr. Stanley was allowed to continue practice within the structure of a rehabilitation plan. She and her husband began couples therapy, and she saw Dr. Ford for long-term individual dynamic therapy. She was deeply devoted to the therapy and determined to avoid any future boundary violations in her career. As noted earlier in the chapter, a fundamental principle of psychodynamic thinking is that multiple factors often converge to produce particular types of behavior. Psychotherapeutic exploration revealed that this basic principle was very much in evidence with Dr. Stanley.
>
> As she reflected on what had happened with Georgia, Dr. Stanley recognized that she over-identified with Georgia. Like her patient, Dr. Stanley had also been dumped by her first husband. She too had felt lost and did not know where to turn. In her therapy, Dr. Stanley recognized that, in essence, she had fallen in love with an image of herself in the form of Georgia, and she was rescuing her lost, desperate, dependent self in the act of breaking boundaries with Georgia. At the same time, she was hoping to elicit from Georgia the love that she did not receive from her parents or her husbands. Many physicians are deeply defended against their own longing for dependency and love, and they give to others as a way of avoiding those painful longings of their own. Hence Dr. Stanley discovered that she was gratifying her own needs while behaving as though she was altruistically attending to the needs of Georgia.
>
> As Dr. Stanley continued to explore the various motives for her attraction to Georgia with Dr. Ford, she recognized that the rescue fantasy with Georgia had overtones of how she had attempted to rescue her mother. She told Dr. Ford that her mother was a "martyr" who was never happy with anything in her life. She seemed to be more miserable than any of the other mothers in her neighborhood. Hence Dr. Stanley spent much of her childhood trying to make her mother feel better, enacting a role reversal—mothering her own mother. She recognized she had unconsciously re-created this with Georgia—in fact, she was both mothering and *receiving* mothering.
>
> Dr. Ford asked Dr. Stanley why she said, "I love you too," after Georgia had told Dr. Stanley that she loved her. This question led to useful reflection on the part of Dr. Stanley. She said she did not ordinarily say this to her patients, as she felt it was not professional. On the other hand, she admitted to a conviction that love itself could be healing. Like many of those who enter the helping professions, Dr. Stanley harbored a secret fantasy that the knowledge of medical tech-

niques was secondary to love and its healing power, despite abundant evidence to the contrary (Gabbard and Lester 2003).

Near the end of her psychotherapy, Dr. Stanley observed that in many ways she had really not known Georgia. She reflected that Georgia was an amalgam of her mother, her disavowed view of herself, and a host of other figures from her past that she had desperately wanted to rescue from despair. She commented on the oft-quoted aphorism that "Love is blind" and told Dr. Ford, with some degree of shame, that she had not been able to realistically assess either the true nature of Georgia's personality nor the consequences of her impaired judgment. She recalled that it never occurred to her that she could find herself in trouble with the licensing board when the relationship began. She felt her love was unimpeachable and that no one could possibly object to it. In the meantime, her couples therapy had greatly improved her relationship with her husband, and they regularly scheduled time together to avoid setting up a vulnerable situation in the future for Dr. Stanley.

Dr. Ford felt warmly toward Dr. Stanley. She viewed her as a competent, dedicated doctor who had a good heart. She found herself feeling protective of her and even wondered if the licensing board had been too harsh with her. As she reflected on her countertransference feelings, she realized that Dr. Stanley's habitual mode of object relatedness involving rescuers and victims had played out in her own therapy in the same way that it had in her treatment of Georgia. She thus recognized her countertransference and avoided criticizing the licensing board or other enactments.

This therapy illustrates only one of many transference-countertransference struggles in the psychotherapy of physicians with a history of sexual boundary violations. Despite the safeguard of confidentiality, the physician-patient may feel that the therapist is really more interested in protecting the public than helping the patient. Therapists may have a corresponding countertransference struggle—namely, they may feel they are policing the profession as much as understanding their patient. Another common problem that arises is that the physician-patient may attempt to re-create an out-of-bounds situation in the therapy similar to the one that created difficulties in the first place. He or she may ask the therapist personal questions, request permission to borrow books from the therapist's office, and try to persuade the therapist to write letters on the patient's behalf (Gabbard 1995b). In addition, the therapist may feel overwhelmed with myriad problems in the physician-patient's world outside the therapy. Marriages crumble. Children become estranged. The medical community may shun the physician-patient. Ancillary treatments may be required. Another common problem, as was the case with Dr. Stanley, is that the patient may feel traumatized by the actions of the licensing board or physicians' health program. As a result, the opening phase of the therapy often involves intense efforts by the physician-patients to make the therapist empathize with their role as victim of the "system." Therapists like Dr. Ford may be quite sympathetic to the physician-patient's feeling of having been treated unfairly.

Psychodynamic Group Therapy

Although most of this chapter has been devoted to individual psychodynamic therapy, the same principles apply to group therapy, and often this modality can be extraordinarily helpful for physicians who are in a crisis. Many specialized residential programs rely on group psychotherapy as a major component, just as chemical dependency programs have historically done.

The group setting offers a number of features that may be useful for physicians, who are often treated in combinations of individual and group approaches. First of all, there is a relief in knowing "I'm not the only one." When a physician can look around the group and see that colleagues who are also suffering can benefit from treatment, the physician may feel a greater sense of optimism about treatment in general. In addition, physicians in a group treatment come to realize that the fact that they have transgressed boundaries, become depressed, made mistakes, or become burned out does not automatically make them a bad person. They see redeeming features in their colleagues and begin to sense that they, too, are redeemable.

Many of the most difficult personality problems that are found in disruptive physicians are best dealt with in dynamic group psychotherapy. A basic axiom of group work is that patients often can take feedback much better from their peers than from the designated therapist. When physicians enter such a group and deny that they have problems or externalize all the difficulties on colleagues, nurses, or the unreasonable nature of licensing boards, they are likely to be confronted by their peers, who can see with penetrating insight that the key issues are being avoided. In one group where a physician who had committed sexual misconduct was voicing his outrage, he blurted out, "The patient seduced *me!* I was the *victim*, not the victimizer. No one seems to understand that." One of his colleagues in the group, who also had engaged in sexual misconduct, retorted bluntly, "I don't care if she took all of her clothes off, it's always the physician's responsibility to act ethically. You can't allow yourself to be seduced." His comment had maximum impact because the colleague had gone through the consequences of sexual boundary violations himself and certainly understood the dynamics of what happened. It was a moment of breakthrough for the patient and led to a turnaround in his treatment.

Finally, groups offer an ideal opportunity to improve one's capacity to mentalize. There will be numerous instances during the course of group session where one member is not thinking about the perspective of others. In group therapy there is a "here and now" opportunity to hear the perspective of others and contrast it with one's own. Moreover, group members can point out to one another when a particular perspective is narrow and does not take into account what others are obviously thinking or seeing.

Key Points

- Psychodynamic psychotherapy is a therapy involving careful attention to the therapist–patient interaction with thoughtfully timed interpretation of transference and resistance. The therapist's countertransference is also a tool that is effectively used to understand what is going on in the patient's other interpersonal relationships.

- Short-term psychodynamic psychotherapy (STPP) lasts 6 months or less, whereas long-term psychodynamic psychotherapy (LTPP) lasts longer and is often open-ended.

- Psychodynamic psychotherapy is really an expressive-supportive therapy in which a therapist shifts flexibly along a continuum of interventions from interpretation on one end to advice and praise on the other.

- Major depression and anxiety disorders, with the exception of obsessive-compulsive disorder, respond well to STPP.

- Cluster C personality disorders and Cluster B personality disorders (with the exception of antisocial personality disorder) are often effectively treated using LTPP.

- Follow-up data suggest that changes continue to occur in an individual after the termination of dynamic psychotherapy.

- Psychological characteristics of the physician must be taken into account in addition to diagnosis when considering whether psychodynamic therapy is indicated.

- Defense mechanisms occur as resistances in dynamic psychotherapy and may require therapeutic work before getting to underlying difficulties.

- Many physicians with borderline and narcissistic personality disorders require a dynamic therapy that focuses on improving the capacity to mentalize.

- Boundary violations are often found to have multiple determinants, so it is misguided to search for one single cause for the boundary transgression.

- Psychodynamic group therapy can be extraordinarily helpful because of unique features of the group.

Individual Cognitive Therapy and Relapse Prevention Treatment

Cognitive-behavioral therapy (CBT) is now recognized as the most heavily researched form of psychotherapy (Wright 2004b). A large number of controlled studies have demonstrated that CBT is an effective treatment for depression, anxiety disorders, and a variety of other conditions (Wright et al. 2006). CBT exists not only as a stand-alone treatment of some conditions but also as an additive treatment to medication in patients with more serious disorders such as refractory depression and bipolar illness. Patients with physical illnesses also respond well to CBT; numerous intervention studies have confirmed its effectiveness in reducing the accompanying anxiety and depression and in improving adherence to treatment, psychosocial adjustment, and quality of life (Sensky 2004).

A brief review of the basic principles of CBT is in order. CBT is derived from a set of principles of cognitive-behavior theory (see Table 9–1) and targets the symptoms and what the patient defines as his or her problems. It is commonly short term, ranging from 5 to 20 sessions depending upon the diagnosis. Each case is conceptualized uniquely according to the patient's history, the diagnostic assessment, clinical observations, and cognitive-behavioral theory. Although the therapeutic relationship shares features of psychodynamic therapy (and other types of psychotherapy), in CBT there is a high degree of collaboration, an

TABLE 9–1.   Key methods of cognitive-behavioral therapy (CBT)

Problem-oriented focus
Individualized case conceptualizations
Collaborative-empirical therapeutic relationship
Socratic questioning
Use of structuring, psychoeducation, and rehearsal to enhance learning
Eliciting and modifying automatic thoughts
Uncovering and changing schemas
Behavioral methods to reverse patterns of helplessness, self-defeating
  behavior, and avoidance
Building CBT skills to help prevent relapse

Source.   Reprinted from Wright JH, Basco MR, Thase ME: *Learning Cognitive-Behavior Therapy.* Washington, DC, American Psychiatric Publishing, 2006. Used with permission.

empirical focus, and action-oriented interventions. Socratic questioning stimulates the patient's curiosity and involves the patient in self-discovery of misperceptions and idiosyncratic thinking. Setting an agenda, explaining key concepts, and educating with prescribed readings and other sources of information are fundamental to the treatment.

Much of CBT helps the patient to identify and change maladaptive automatic thoughts and schemas (Wright et al. 2006). The therapy includes keeping a record of thoughts, pinpointing cognitive errors, examining the evidence, reattribution (modifying attributional style), listing rational alternatives, and cognitive rehearsal. This process takes repeated practice, some with the therapist but most outside the therapy setting. Another key feature of CBT is the bidirectional relationship with behavior. Change in thinking results in changed behavior and vice versa. As patients improve by gaining skills of cognitive self-mastery and changing maladaptive behaviors, they reduce the risk of relapse. In the face of stress and possible triggers of symptom return, they now are equipped to identify automatic thoughts or patterns and to enact rehearsal techniques to cope more effectively.

Applicability to Physician-Patients

There are many reasons why CBT is an important therapeutic modality in the treatment of symptomatic physicians:

- Depression and anxiety disorders are not uncommon in doctors, so ill physicians are subject to the same cognitive errors as the rest of humankind. Some of these are absolutistic (all or none) thinking, magnification and minimization, personalization, and catastrophic thinking (Wright et al. 2003). Whether depressed, anxious, or both, physicians presenting for treatment may be demoralized, self-absorbed, and reduced in their cognitive ability to solve problems and complete tasks both at work and in their personal lives.

- Some physicians prefer therapy to medication, or they may be completely against the use of medication for the treatment of anxiety or depression. Even when the treating clinician believes that both are required, CBT is an appropriate initial choice of treatment. If gains are minimal with CBT, the use of medication can be revisited later.

- Many physicians like the parameters of CBT. It is relatively time-efficient in duration, and this appeals to the busy doctor who wants to get well quickly. Physicians who are not psychodynamically oriented may like the fact that the focus is on the specifics of one's current life situation. Because the theory and application of CBT is problem-oriented, this is in keeping with the training and everyday practice of clinicians. Most important, crafting a plan of action with the therapist engages the physician in an intellectual exercise that offers early relief from feelings of helplessness and hopelessness and a restoration of control, which is fundamental in the personality makeup of most physicians.

- CBT requires a type of therapist–patient relationship that interests most physicians because it is interactive, straightforward, and mutually engaging. Because the treatment is pragmatic and emphasizes self-monitoring and bidirectional feedback, the physician-patient who has tended to view psychiatry as esoteric or confusing will feel at ease. Structuring principles of CBT, such agenda-setting at the beginning of each session and assigning homework, resonates with the "student" persona in physicians regardless of age and stage of professional life.

- Psychoeducation is a basic element in CBT. Being lifelong learners, physicians—especially when living with a phobia of some sort or struggling with depression—are hungry for an explanation of what is wrong with them and what can be done to alleviate their symptoms. They are open to explanations, answers to questions, and reading materials (Basco 1999; Burns 1999; Greenberger and Padesky 1995; Wright and Basco 2001).

  Computer-assisted programming is a promising and evolving application of CBT (Wright 2004a). Among its many advantages are improved access to treatment, reliability and effectiveness, and emphasis on self-help. After traveling for an initial face-to-face assessment by a clinician, physicians who practice in rural and remote areas could benefit tremendously from this type of ongoing treatment.

- Many physicians have alcoholism or other forms of drug abuse or dependence. Behavioral, cognitive-behavioral, and motivational treatments are among the most well-defined and rigorously studied psychotherapeutic interventions for substance use disorders (Carroll et al. 2004). They are effective across a range of substance abuse, including alcohol, stimulants, opioids, and cannabis. They are applicable in a variety of clinical settings and in conjunction with medications such as naltrexone and disulfiram.

- CBT is helpful in other illnesses that befall physicians and bring them to psychiatric attention. Cognitive distortions are rife in physicians with eating disorders, especially anorexia nervosa. Bulimic physicians may respond to behavioral techniques that examine more adaptive eating. Physicians hospitalized for psychotic illnesses—especially mania and delusional depression—will respond to cognitive techniques aimed at medication adherence, self-destructive and self-referential thinking, grandiosity, and shame. Physicians with personality disorders can also be helped with CBT. Beck and Freeman (1990) pointed out that individuals with personality disorders have idiosyncratic cognitions in four main areas: basic beliefs, view of self, view of others, and strategies for social interaction. Treatment is longer than that for anxiety or depression and requires the therapist to set firm but reasonable limits. Physicians with borderline personality disorder, especially those with self-destructive and suicidal behaviors, can be helped with dialectical behavior therapy (Linehan 1993a).

- Physicians with medical disorders who are referred to mental health professionals for associated psychiatric conditions can also be helped with CBT. The list of such medical disorders is long and includes fibromyalgia, chronic fatigue syndrome, chronic pain, rheumatoid arthritis, inflammatory bowel disease, multiple sclerosis, hypertension, obesity, diabetes, and more. Strategies are aimed at minimizing catastrophic thinking, stabilizing emotions, and coping with the narcissistic injury attached to medical vulnerability and reduced level of function in physicians.

The following case is an example of a young physician who, in addition to having a complicated grief reaction after the death of a parent, presented with phobic avoidance of a medical board examination. It illustrates how CBT strategies, specifically exposure therapy and cognitive restructuring, were helpful for amelioration of his symptoms and resulted in a successful outcome.

Case Example

Dr. Chambers is a 29-year-old resident in oncology who consulted a psychiatrist 2 months after his father hanged himself. Dr. Chambers was struggling with extreme loss and guilt that he had not intervened in some way to prevent his father's death. Despite supportive psychotherapy, his symptoms worsened. He developed early morning wakening, severe fatigue, short-term memory difficulty, and weight loss. Antidepressant medication was helpful in ameliorating his vegetative symptoms, and he began to cope better with his grief. At this point, he disclosed to his psychiatrist that he had just deferred a set of medical examinations that he had initially failed 24 months earlier when he began his residency. Probing revealed that this was the third round of examinations he had studied intensively for and cancelled. "I can't explain it. When I failed the first set I was humiliated. I had never failed an exam in my life. But I understood why I failed because I wasn't prepared. I was worrying about my dad because he was getting really depressed then, he had attempted suicide, and I took a few weeks off to be with him after he was discharged from the psych unit. But then I put my nose to the grindstone and studied hard. I knew my stuff, but a few days before I just panicked and called the examination office and asked for a deferral. This has happened three times now."

Dr. Chambers was given a diagnosis of social phobia by his psychiatrist based on the criteria of marked and persistent fear of a performance situation that involved scrutiny (the qualifying general medical examination) with accompanying humiliation from his earlier failure of the examination; exposure to the feared situation caused anxiety; subjective recognition by Dr. Chambers that his fear of failure was excessive; and avoidance of the repeat examination that interfered with his career progression. Dr. Chambers was open to treatment that included both exposure therapy and cognitive restructuring. With regard to the former, he and his psychiatrist constructed a hierarchy of his fears around the examination. In classic fashion, this ranged all the way from imagining the examination several weeks ahead to actually driving to the examination site and walking into the building. Dr. Chambers easily identified his anxiety symptoms (increased heart rate, sweaty palms, flushing and nausea) and was able to develop a self-rating numerical system. Having practiced yoga on and off since college, he had no difficulty "reading" bodily signals of arousal and tension. Deep and slow breathing calmed him immediately, and he advanced quickly to successive stages of practice. In a very short time, he could face the examination with much less anticipatory anxiety.

With regard to cognitive restructuring, Dr. Chambers was able to see that his fear of failure was irrational. He had failed only one examination in his life, and that exam took place in the midst of overwhelming family stress. He needed to be reminded of his stellar academic performance in the past. Regarding his humiliation, he came to see that this was an excessive self-judgment and not shared by his family members and close friends. In a purely logical way, he was also able to accept that he had adequately prepared for the repeat examination, that the preparation was standard historically for him and that there was no rational reason why he should fail again. With cognitive therapy he easily saw how avoidance reduced his anxiety only in the short term and that the longer he avoided the next set of examinations, the more entrenched this would become. He also responded to the notion of relief—that it would feel good to put the examination behind him, free up some time in his very busy life, and move forward with an avocation he yearned to do. This was to take up the saxophone again and join a local amateur jazz band at the medical center. He set this up as a reward. Everything went well, and he passed the examination with ease.

The combination of exposure therapy and cognitive restructuring is known to be helpful in patients with social anxiety disorder. Dr. Chambers was an ideal candidate not only because of his symptoms but also because of his intelligence and high degree of motivation to conquer the problem. He practiced diligently in his efforts to reduce his anticipatory anxiety toward the feared situation, and he worked hard with his psychiatrist to examine his distorted and irrational thinking about failure. He was also "fed up" with his problem and was very keen to get beyond passing the examination and have time freed up for personal pursuits.

The next case example illustrates how agoraphobia in a physician prevented her from driving unaccompanied to appointments with her psychiatrist. She had a morbid fear of developing a panic attack despite never having had one. This fear was extreme and reinforced her avoidance. She was treated with exposure therapy and reevaluation of her catastrophic thinking.

Case Example

Dr. Wise is a 50-year-old physician who had a very limited private practice. Because of residual symptoms of her bipolar illness, she was only able to work about 20 hours per week. She was very compliant with her medication, which included a mood stabilizer, antidepressant, and second-generation neuroleptic. She had only been hospitalized once in the past for a manic episode that occurred shortly after she completed her residency. The psychotherapy that she had received over the years had been mainly supportive (individual) in type, although she had had a course of conjoint marital therapy for her marriage that ended in divorce 10 years ago. Because her psychiatrist, who practiced in the same medical building as she did, was retiring, he referred her to a new psychiatrist who worked at the medical school in the closest urban setting, some 30 miles away. Her opening words were "I have agoraphobia—I can't drive downtown to see you—I'll get a panic attack and kill someone—it's too congested and noisy here—my next door neighbor drove me today. Do you do telephone appointments so that I don't need to see you again?"

The psychiatrist obtained a more detailed history from Dr. Wise to ascertain specifics about her agoraphobia. Interestingly, Dr. Wise had never had a panic attack. However, she was terrified of having one for two reasons. First, her mother had had panic attacks for a number of years while Dr. Wise was growing up. Dr. Wise had no sympathy: "Mom was a drama queen; she used her anxiety attacks to manipulate my dad and us kids. When I was in medical school and learned about them and how frightening they can be, I immediately felt guilty—and I still do. How insensitive of me." Second, Dr. Wise had treated a number of patients with panic disorder in her work as an emergency physician. She had had no difficulty empathizing with their intense psychological distress.

Dr. Wise responded nicely to a combination of exposure therapy and reevaluation of her catastrophic thinking about panic attacks. However, the initial visits were difficult. Dr. Wise was very talkative and digressive, but she had no insight into this. When gently confronted by her psychiatrist that his approach involved focus and structure, she felt hurt and offended. "My last psychiatrist never interrupted me like you do. He gave me the entire hour to talk about whatever I wanted. And that was very helpful." When her current psychiatrist explained the difference between supportive psychotherapy and cognitive-behavioral therapy, Dr. Wise felt much better. However, it took a while before therapy time was used efficiently, agenda items were addressed as planned, and a truly collaborative process was in place. This process involved considerable patience on the part of the psychiatrist.

Dr. Wise had studied and was interested in exposure therapy. She had already told her neighbor, Fay, about her problem. Fay was not only very understanding but also willing to help Dr. Wise overcome her difficulty driving into the urban core of the city. Dr. Wise practiced relaxation exercises before and during driving, initially in her suburban neighborhood and gradually working her way closer to the city. They started at quieter times of the day and enhanced these driving trips by playing CDs that Dr. Wise found soothing. Conjuring up beautiful vistas helped her (Dr. Wise was very outdoorsy, feeling most serene walking on the beach and hiking in the mountains). Before they increased the distance from home toward the city, Dr. Wise repeated the same journey alone until she could master a prescribed set point. Both Fay and the psychiatrist reinforced Dr. Wise's successes and challenged her tendency to belittle her gains.

Tackling catastrophic thinking involved discussing the probability of her having a panic attack. She was able to accept that she had lived 50 years without one and that chances were slim that she would have one now. The psychiatrist directed her away from her guilt about not helping her mother (a negative experience) to her success at helping her emergency department patients with panic disorder (a positive experience). Borrowing a psychodynamic term, he used the notion of "observing ego" and urged her to immediately employ her helpful professional skills for herself if (in the rare likelihood) she should become panicky. Dr. Wise liked this, and it reinforced her sense of autonomy and ability to help herself. They also discussed her original fear of getting a panic attack and killing someone. Dr. Wise started to laugh and said, "Come to think of it, of the many patients I've treated in the ER over my career with panic attacks, I don't recall any one of them killing anyone. Or even hurting anyone. But almost all of them have verbalized the same fear as me!" She went on: "You know what? Except for the tunnel and the one bridge that I have to navigate on my way here to your office, I can always pull my car over to the side and get control of myself. I'm already dealing with the tunnel and the bridge by paying attention to my breathing, opening the window a bit for fresh air, and listening to my CD. And those strategies work."

It was well into her treatment that Dr. Wise "confessed" that she always carried one or two 1-mg sublingual lorazepam tablets with her. These were self-prescribed, and she had never used one. In fact, she wondered if they were still effective, with the tablets having long exceeded their expiration date 6 years earlier. She proudly told her psychiatrist how far she had come: "When I first began driving toward the city without Fay in the car I had my lorazepam tablet sitting out on the dashboard, all ready to be popped under my tongue at a moment's notice. As I got better and better at driving the same distance, I put it in my pocket so it was no longer visible. Then I put it in my purse. And that's where it sits today. I'm not ready to toss it yet but maybe someday." Her psychiatrist thanked her for telling him this story, reiterated how hard she was working in therapy, and congratulated her on her achievements.

This case illustrates how effective exposure therapy can be in someone who is highly motivated to overcome her difficulty. There was minimal secondary gain in remaining symptomatic and so much more for her to gain psychologically in developing mastery over her symptoms. As an emergency physician, she was used to being in control, especially when she was very busy and multitasking with several sick patients at once. She hated being dependent on her friend to accompany her in driving the car out of her neighborhood. Engaging with her psychiatrist in a mutual process of understanding her illogical thoughts about panicking and harming others really appealed to her, and she worked hard at this. Because she tended to minimize her improvement, she also benefited from the modeling effect of positive affirmations from her psychiatrist and his exhortations that she praise herself more.

The next example is that of a physician with both social anxiety disorder and depression. He was terrified to speak up at grand rounds. His psychiatrist used the two CBT strategies of examining the evidence and de-catastrophizing, which are known to be helpful in this disorder (Wright et al. 2006).

Case Example

Dr. Ellis is a 42-year-old hematologist who consulted a psychiatrist shortly after accepting an academic position in a new city. He cited the geographical move as one of his major stressors in addition to his wife's first pregnancy and their long struggle with infertility. His symptoms included worry that he might not be able to meet the demands of the job and a feeling of fraudulence that he got the job in the first place. "I think I've got that impostor syndrome that I've read about in women physicians. I feel like I've fooled my department head and any day now she will call me into her office and say 'the jig is up.'" Dr. Ellis also had middle insomnia, with obsessive ruminating at night and lots of fatigue through the day. He had gained 10 pounds of weight and hated the way he looked. "I can't stop berating myself. I'm not a good doctor, I'm fat, I'm not a good husband, and I'm not confident about what kind of father I'm going to be." He had diagnosed panic attacks in himself and was self-medicating with a beta blocker medication.

His psychiatrist diagnosed major depressive disorder and prescribed an antidepressant medication. This relieved many of his symptoms. In his third visit with the psychiatrist, he talked about a longstanding inability to speak up at grand rounds and ask questions. This began when he was an intern, and he had trouble on bedside rounds. He would lose his voice or it would crack. He could not breathe and became self-conscious and embarrassed. This made him more anxious and panicky. He started to think of ways to avoid presenting cases to others. On two occasions he called in sick when he was scheduled to give grand rounds, despite weeks of preparation and practicing at home in front of a mirror. He admitted that he felt very handicapped by his symptoms. His psychiatrist diagnosed social anxiety disorder and recommended CBT in addition to the antidepressant medication.

Because Dr. Ellis was obtaining good relief from much of his anxiety by the specific type of antidepressant that he was taking, he was treated with CBT—specifically, examining the evidence and de-catastrophizing. Examining the evidence works against automatic thoughts. Dr. Ellis and his psychiatrist listed evidence for and against the validity of his automatic thoughts, evaluated this evidence, and then worked on changing his thinking to be consistent with the newfound evidence. This approach was applied both in the office and as a homework assignment for Dr. Ellis. The "evidence for" list was short: his voice had cracked when he was an intern 15 years ago, he was new to the city, and he had not earned a position of certainty yet at this medical center. The "evidence against" list was longer: he was a Phi Beta Kappa in college and a gold medalist at his medical school; so far, no one had concluded that he earned his degrees fraudulently; it was 15 years since his internship, and he could not remember his voice cracking more than once; he acknowledged that after two decades of attending grand rounds he could not recall anyone berating someone for asking a stupid or inappropriate question; on most occasions in rounds he did have the correct answer or was about to ask a very important question that was posed within minutes by a colleague; and he had given rounds twice in the past 6 years, both of which were well received. (Dr. Ellis, in his understated and self-critical way, had trouble accepting laudatory remarks after his rounds and attempted to diminish the authenticity of positive feedback because he had taken a beta blocker before the experience.)

After evaluating the evidence, Dr. Ellis worked very hard at raising his hand at rounds. He found it easier if he sat near the front of the auditorium, listened carefully to the presenter, and the moment that the presenter finished and called for questions, he threw his hand in the air. This gave him less time to get more anxious as others asked questions before him and diminished the fear that someone might "steal his question" by asking it first. He also realized how easy it was to relax once he posed his question, especially if the presenter prefaced his answer with something positive like "That's a great question, thanks for asking it."

Regarding de-catastrophizing, Dr. Ellis' psychiatrist asked him, "What's the worst thing that could happen when you ask a question at rounds or have to present grand rounds?" Dr. Ellis responded with the following: "Nothing will come out of my mouth, I'll be mute. Or I will stammer and stutter. Then my colleagues will stare at me and I will get flushed, if I'm not blushing already. If I can get the words out, I don't think that they will laugh at me or think that I'm a stupid hematologist. I think I've moved beyond that." Through discussion, Dr. Ellis was able to see that the likelihood of these possibilities was small and that even if they did happen he could cover by stating "Sorry, I've got a bit of a cold" or "Let me start again" as well as taking a deep breath. Having this plan helped him gain confidence.

Dr. Ellis signed up to present some of his recent research at a grand rounds 8 weeks away. At the suggestion of his psychiatrist, he considered joining Toastmasters. This international resource was of help to him both online (www. toastmasters.org) and locally. He joined a club and got to practice public speaking well before his scheduled rounds. In a session after his very successful presentation, Dr. Ellis reported that he was delighted with how he conducted himself as well as the oral feedback after the rounds and the written evaluations.

This case illustrates the effectiveness of these two CBT strategies in a physician who understands the historical underpinnings of his symptoms but who also knows that years have passed since they began. He knew "intellectually" that he was not stupid and that, as an associate professor, he had merit in his field. He was also willing to push himself and had a "game plan" if his voice failed him. The successful experiences of asking the first question when the speaker finished (and being commended for being erudite) and presenting his own research at grand rounds lessened his fear and boosted his confidence markedly.

Here is an example of a very obsessional physician who was severely ill at the time of consultation with both a mood and anxiety disorder and who was unable to remain on psychotropic medications of any sort because of intolerable side effects. He was a good candidate for CBT, and the psychiatrist examined cognitive errors (Beck et al. 1979) with him. This, combined with a respectful therapeutic alliance, helped him to regain his health.

Case Example

Dr. Perry is a 38-year-old radiologist who was referred to a psychiatrist by a concerned colleague who reached out to him when she found him crying in his office. He was a "no show" for a scheduled interventional procedure, and she had gone to find him, but for several weeks prior to this incident she had been worried about him because he was not his usual self. Dr. Perry began the visit like this: "I'm a mental health mess and a treatment failure. I've seen two previous psychiatrists and nothing has worked. I can't take medication, period. They have tried antidepressants, tranquilizers, and anticonvulsants. Pediatric doses give me very unpleasant—no, crippling—side effects so severe that I won't even try any kind of medication, in any form, of any type." When the psychiatrist invited Dr. Perry to describe his symptoms, Dr. Perry said: "I've got cervical pain that nobody, including myself, can understand. All investigations are normal and I've had the works. But I suffer constantly. This makes me anxious and sends my mood into a nosedive. I'm a perfectionist, an OC [obsessive-compulsive] type. I can't sleep—the pain drives me nuts. I don't normally cry but I do now. I'm not sad, I'm frustrated and very worried that I'll never get better. My appetite is off. I've lost almost 15 pounds over the past 2 months. I've aged a decade in the last 3 to 4 months. I don't have the energy that I normally have. It's all going into worry. I can't turn my mind off. It's hard to do my work because I can't focus. I'm afraid of screwing up and harming someone. Last week I noticed that my memory is going. I can't remember what I read, and I'm afraid that someone might quiz me. Medical journals freak me out because I can't process—even the abstracts. I'm convinced I'm developing Alzheimer's. I've even become a bit of a homebody; I'm nervous to go food shopping alone. I said 'no' to a movie last night because I'm kind of afraid of getting trapped in the theater. It's all becoming doom and gloom as each day goes on. Last night I paced back and forth in my living room—why, I don't know; it was sort of beyond my control—I just had to do it."

The psychiatrist concluded that Dr. Perry was very ill and considered (on Axis I) major depressive disorder, generalized anxiety disorder, and somatoform disorder. On Axis II, he diagnosed obsessive-compulsive traits. Dr. Perry was placed on medical leave, which was a relief to him. Because he was unable to tolerate medication of any kind and he was not acutely suicidal on detailed risk assessment, his psychiatrist discussed CBT with him. Although his thinking was negative and pessimistic about any form of treatment, Dr. Perry was guardedly open to treatment. They started with cognitive errors. There were several of these: selective abstraction and arbitrary inference (Dr. Perry jumped to conclusions with little information in a highly subjective way, e.g., a self-diagnosis of Alzheimer's); magnification (his preoccupation with medication side effects; he concluded that he was a treatment failure and that he would never get better); and catastrophic thinking (his grim prognosis for himself did not include the possibility that another psychiatrist might be able to help and that psychopharmacology is only one treatment approach). Dr. Perry liked the cognitive theme of the work with his psychiatrist: "You treat me like a person with a brain. Even though I've lost my intellectual prowess, I feel like we are working together on this. Thanks."

Dr. Perry came to understand how maladaptive his thinking had become. For example, he began to see that his underlying perfectionistic personality that is so common in physicians and that enables them to thrive in medicine was in many ways working against him. He could not tolerate symptoms that did not easily go away or respond to medication. In fact, symptoms terrified him: "What's next? Hallucinations and talking to myself at ward rounds? Being on a locked unit?" As a doctor, he now felt inadequate, dangerous, and like a failure. He also felt he had failed as a patient. Most important, he concluded that he no longer had control over his life. His psychiatrist worked closely with him trying to help him understand alternate ways of looking at himself and his symptoms. This included pointing out constantly ways in which Dr. Perry was still in charge and reminding him of his strengths and autonomy. Dr. Perry came to accept that his lowered self-esteem was new and temporary, that prior to his illness his self-esteem was adequate if not better than adequate. He was very hurt by complaints from his girlfriend and medical colleagues that he was "totally into himself and no longer cared about anyone else." His psychiatrist helped him to understand that morbid egocentricity is common in depression and leaves when the person is well again. The same approach was used to address his pervasive sense of hopelessness and blighted morale.

Keeping a detailed record of his thoughts, identifying errors and automatic thinking, and recording more adaptive thoughts did not appeal to Dr. Perry. He felt that it reinforced his obsessive-compulsive nature and made him feel worse: "more anal, more screwed up than I am already." However, he was open to simple journaling, with no pressure to write every day or about what to write. This worked nicely because he felt more in control. He made entries only when he could start with a positive change and some smidgen of hope. He carried his journal with him at all times, along with his digital camera. His psychiatrist suggested that he take a photograph whenever he felt moved or touched by something. This reinforced the idea that he could still appreciate beauty in his environment. At times he brought some photos into a therapy session. The humanistic response of his psychiatrist to pictures of children at play in the park, a seagull in flight, a bright orange sunset, and more was pivotal. This interaction highlighted Dr. Perry's relational being, reminded him of how much he was a key player in his treatment, and significantly divested him of much of his negative self-absorption.

Dr. Perry responded well to CBT but over an extended time line. He remained off work for almost a year. Once his mood lifted somewhat and his anxiety lessened, he was able to engage in other forms of psychotherapy. Psychodynamically oriented psychotherapy addressed unresolved early childhood issues that needed uncovering and working through, especially the first and second divorces of each of his parents that occurred while he was growing up. He developed an interest in group therapy that was conducted by a local psychologist and began this process at the time that he discontinued treatment with his psychiatrist. Interestingly, one of the appealing dimensions of the group was that it was insight oriented and comprised exclusively of highly educated professional men and women.

This case illustrates the benefits of CBT with a highly anxious, discouraged, and somewhat isolated physician. His symptoms terrified him, so working on his cognitive errors was salutary. Reframing hurtful criticisms of himself (his selfish preoccupation) and psychoeducation helped him to understand what unrelenting psychiatric symptoms can do to one's morale and world view. His efforts to capture positive experiences—whether an achievement to be entered in his journal or a photograph of a happy or beautiful moment—came to replace and eclipse much of his exaggerated and negative thinking. His mood and behavior improved with his changed thinking. Dr. Perry's case also illustrates how different types of therapy can be complementary and work synergistically to add breadth and depth to the treatment plan. Many patients who benefit from brief CBT wish to go on to explore unconscious conflicts in dynamic psychotherapy.

Biofeedback and Relaxation Therapy

Although not strictly CBT strategies, biofeedback and relaxation therapy can be used with CBT in the treatment of symptomatic physicians. *Biofeedback* is a type of behavioral medicine approach that registers and displays physiological signals to the patient with various ailments that have a tensional component. People are taught to recognize simple forms of bodily function and to learn ways of controlling abnormal patterns. A physician with intermittent, but otherwise benign, hypertension might benefit from biofeedback.

Relaxation therapy is defined by its name. It may be initiated in the psychiatrist's office, but it is then practiced at home. The patient contracts and relaxes various muscle groups while seated in a comfortable chair. This is often coupled with visualizing a very pleasant scene and focusing on this. There are many commercially produced relaxation tapes that individuals listen to at home. Some physicians use them at noon to counteract the stress of their morning's work and to prepare for the afternoon.

TABLE 9–2.   Beliefs about substance abuse

- I don't have any control over craving.
- Once it starts, the only way to cope with craving is to use.
- I've passed the point of no return—I'll never be able to stop drinking.
- You need willpower not to drink, and I don't have it.
- I can't have fun without getting high.
- It doesn't matter if I stop using—no one cares.
- I can't cope without drinking.
- My life is already ruined—and I might as well get high.
- No one can push me around—I'll quit when I'm ready.

Source.   Reprinted from Thase ME: "Cognitive-Behavioral Therapy for Substance Abuse," in *American Psychiatric Press Review of Psychiatry,* Vol. 16. Edited by Dickstein LJ, Riba MB, Oldham JM. Washington, DC, American Psychiatric Press, 1997, pp. 45–71. Copyright 1997, American Psychiatric Press. Used with permission.

Relapse Prevention Treatment

Relapse prevention therapy is grounded in the theory that relapse (a return to previous behaviors) occurs when a patient who has insufficient ways of coping is confronted with a high-risk situation, problem, or emotional state (Berkowitz 2003). When applied to the addictions (both chemical and nonchemical), relapse prevention therapy involves strategies and techniques to enhance self-control and foster abstinence (Marlatt and Gordon 1985). These include self-monitoring to recognize false beliefs and drug cravings; identification of situations in which one is at high risk for substance use (especially negative emotional states, interpersonal conflicts, and social pressure); and development of strategies for avoiding or coping with affects or situations that stimulate drug craving.

There are many beliefs relevant to the onset and maintenance of substance use disorders (Thase 1997) as noted in Table 9–2. An important piece of the CBT model is to help the patient recognize that urges and cravings to drink alcohol or to use drugs are often associated with relevant beliefs about drug or alcohol abuse. In addition to situational cues, such as driving past a bar or seeing an advertisement on TV, urges and cravings can be triggered by daydreams, memories, and most especially dysphoric emotions like anger, anxiety, sadness, or boredom. What is key is to anticipate problems that one might meet in recovery and to know how to prevent recurrence.

Motivational enhancement therapy, or motivational interviewing, is a relatively new approach that addresses the patient's level of motivation (Miller and

Rollnick 2002). It is grounded in a motivational "stages of change" model. Because poor motivation to change is not uncommon in the addictions, it is particularly applicable here. Physicians who are unmotivated (precontemplation stage) or have a lot of ambivalence about changing whatever their problem behavior is (contemplation stage) may derive a lot of benefit from motivational enhancement therapy. Once they have made a commitment to some specific action plan for change, they are ready to benefit from relapse prevention.

Physicians who have been charged with sexual offenses and are undergoing treatment for compulsive sexual behavior (or paraphilias) can benefit from relapse prevention therapy. Indeed relapse prevention is currently the most popular cognitive-behavioral approach to treating sex offenders (Laws et al. 2000). This is an ever-evolving field that includes "risk assessment" as a conceptual framework paired with the skills training "modules" of dialectical behavior therapy (Linehan 1993b) into an integrated approach called recidivism risk reduction therapy (Wheeler et al. 2005). This therapy can be useful for physicians who are receiving treatment in both residential and ambulatory settings, especially those utilizing a group therapy format.

Relapse prevention therapy is applicable beyond the addictions. It is also useful for patients struggling with anorexia nervosa (accepting and maintaining the weight that has been regained with vigorous treatment programs) and mood disorders (motivational enhancement around the advantages and disadvantages of continuing to take antidepressant medication). Although most physicians, including psychiatrists, have an intellectual grasp of the importance of remaining on essential and mood-enhancing medications to keep their symptoms at bay, when they become patients they really are little different than lay people. Relapse prevention therapy greatly increases pharmacotherapy treatment adherence in doctors.

Here is an example of a physician in recovery for substance dependence who, in addition to 12-Step recovery, was treated with relapse prevention techniques. With the help of his psychiatrist, he recognized and articulated emotional states and other pressures that put him at risk for relapse. He also learned effective methods of coping with affect and situations, which gave him mastery over his disease.

Case Example

When Dr. Jamison consulted his psychiatrist he was already in recovery for cocaine dependence. He had started using the drug shortly after he completed his residency and began making a lot of money. His addiction was severely entrenched when he first attended Narcotics Anonymous. He was assessed by a physician health program in his area and was sent away to a treatment center. He had had two relapses and two readmissions to treatment centers when he requested psychiatric consultation. He wondered if he needed something more than what he felt was excellent 12-Step recovery treatment, and he had several questions: "Do I have bipolar illness? Is my wife correct that I have adult ADD? Is it the stress of my job? I'm a transplant surgeon, and it's very demanding. I'm so afraid of another relapse. Do I need psychoanalysis or hypnosis? Maybe I was abused by my mother or father and I've repressed it and I used cocaine to cope?"

Dr. Jamison was thoroughly assessed by his psychiatrist and not found to have any other diagnoses except substance dependence, but he was terrified of using cocaine again. Relapse prevention therapy was suggested to him by his psychiatrist, who asked "What are the qualities that make you so good at your work?" Dr. Jamison replied: "Well I'm very task oriented. I like to think my way through a problem in a very logical and methodical way. I love a challenge. And I've got lots of energy to get the job done." "Maybe we can use some of these things to keep you clean and sober," replied his doctor.

Because of Dr. Jamison's eagerness for help, his psychiatrist was able to use a number of techniques that are the hallmark of motivational therapy for the addictions (Carroll et al. 2004). These included asking open-ended questions, making affirmative comments, using reflective statements, employing summary responses, giving personal feedback, eliciting self-motivational statements, and constructing a plan for change. He was doing quite a lot of reading on addictions, and although he tended toward intellectualization, he was very curious about all of the interacting variables—unpleasant mood states and stimuli, automatic thinking, urges and cravings, and vulnerability to drug use. He was very open about his profound emotions regarding cocaine: "Just talking about cocaine makes me crazy. I think of how crappy I felt when I'd get the urge to use. Then the high I got racing off to my dealer. The adrenaline rush even before I snorted. But I haven't forgotten the emotional and physiological aftermath. The self-loathing. How pathetic I felt. The shame. And now the risks: losing my medical license, my wife and kids, and my unbelievably compassionate colleagues at work. No…I can't do it again…ever."

Dr. Jamison worked hard at naming the emotions that made him most frightened and that were linked with drug use in the past. These included emotions that resulted in his overuse of alcohol while in college and medical school. Boredom was one; he had daydreamed a lot during lectures and escaped into fantasy. Restlessness was another, with a need for physical movement. He had little tolerance for sadness or despondency and knew that he tended to suppress these feelings: "I blame my mother for this; she was a miserable, self-pitying martyr who wouldn't smile even if she won the lottery." Another emotion was anger. "I stuff my anger, except when I'm playing hockey. Then I let it rip. I don't play anymore. I associate hockey with drinking beer afterwards. Can't do that now." Fatigue was also a trigger because this led to feelings of entitlement: "I've worked hard today; this was a tough case. My liver transplant will save this boy's life. I'm tired. I deserve to get high."

Conceiving and practicing adaptive ways of coping with dysphoric mood states was a major piece of his relapse prevention therapy. This reinforced the 12-Step principles of his recovery program. He cut back on the number of hours he worked per week, and his partners were very accepting of this. He brought lunches and other snacks to work to avoid protracted hunger (another trigger). He joined a gym and took up karate. He signed up for a course in scuba diving. With his wife's assistance, they scheduled "dates" together on the family calendar. For a long time, he avoided the downtown core of his city because of its association with drug dealing. Most important, he came to accept that mild and evanescent feelings of depression—and sadness—are okay and normal feeling states. They are not feelings of weakness or self-pity.

Dr. Jamison responded nicely to treatment. He was highly motivated to remain abstinent and knew the adverse consequences he would face if he relapsed. He left with more recognition of important emotions and armed with adaptive strategies to handle them. He remained actively involved in his 12-Step recovery program.

Key Points

- CBT is a well-researched and effective treatment for many types of psychiatric illness.

- Because physicians are lifelong learners, many doctors with mood and anxiety disorders are interested in CBT. The collaborative nature of the work and its emphasis on thinking and behavioral change are appealing. Because of the ambivalence that many symptomatic physicians have toward taking psychotropic medication, CBT as an adjunct to or instead of drug treatment (when appropriate) has great acceptance.

- Similarly, physicians who are not dynamically oriented may find CBT of interest because of its problem-centered focus and pragmatic interventions.

- Several case examples of physicians with a range of symptoms and diagnoses are described and their treatment with CBT is outlined.

- Relapse prevention treatment is an especially important type of CBT that is very applicable to addictions in physicians, both chemical and nonchemical. It is an important modality of treatment for eating disorders in doctors and can be very helpful in improving pharmacotherapy compliance in physicians living with mood disorders.

Couples in Conflict and Their Treatment

The challenges of the medical marriage are well known and have been documented in the literature since the 1970s in many oft-cited articles and books (Coombs 1971; Derdeyn 1978; Fine 1981; Fletcher and Fletcher 1993; Gabbard and Menninger 1988; Garvey and Tuason 1979; Gerber 1983; Miles et al. 1975; Myers 1994; Notman and Nadelson 1973; Rose and Rosow 1972; Sobecks et al. 1999; Sotile and Sotile 2000; Verlander 2004). Several authors have described personality characteristics that physicians bring to their marriages—characteristics that give their relationships a unique cast and that may both cause and protect against problems (see Ellis and Inbody 1988; Gabbard 1985; Gabbard and Menninger 1989; Myers 1984; Nadelson and Notman 1988; Vaillant et al. 1972).

There are no empirically rigorous studies of marital symptoms and other conflict indices in doctors. There has been no study of rates of help-seeking in physicians with troubled marriages. There is no research that addresses variables such as race, ethnicity, gender, sexual orientation, International Medical Graduate versus United States Medical Graduate, medical specialty, or number of marriage (first, second, or more). Marital therapy outcome studies are scant. Those that do exist are rather old and lack methodological sophistication. Some show good results (Glick and Borus 1984; Goldberg 1975), whereas others reveal less favorable results (Krell and Miles 1976).

Although there are no data on the prevalence of marital problems in doctors, there are some data on divorce, albeit mixed. Doherty and Burge (1989) reported that divorce rates in doctors are lower than in other occupational groups. In contrast, Sotile and Sotile (2000) described divorce rates among doctors as 10%–20% higher than those in the general population. Rollman et al. (1997) studied divorce according to medical specialty, using the Johns Hopkins Precursors Study, but their results are limited by examining only physicians who entered medical school between 1944 and 1960 and by reporting on a narrowly restricted population (i.e., those doctors from one medical school).

It is wise to remember that divorce rates are only one index of marital strain and demise. Many unhappily married physicians never separate. If they do, they may not get divorced and therefore never appear as a statistic. It is sometimes alleged that women physicians have higher divorce rates than male physicians, but to our knowledge, there is no evidence-based research to support this. Even if their rates of divorce are higher, it may reflect the fate of dual career marriages in general (vs. traditional marriages) wherein highly educated and financially independent women do not need to remain in loveless, emotionally empty or abusive relationships. Divorce for at least some physicians is necessary, emotionally affirming, and maybe even lifesaving (e.g., escaping from domestic violence).

Given the cultural mosaic of North American physicians, their marriages are far from monolithic. Although married physicians with troubled relationships constitute the largest group requesting couples therapy, there are many others who seek help. Some physicians are not married but have been in a committed relationship with someone for an indefinite period of time and are encountering problems. They may or may not be cohabiting. One partner may be married, but to someone else—he or she has been separated for some time but is not yet divorced. Some physician couples are in a long-standing intimate and committed relationship that simulates a marriage, but for many reasons, neither partner wants the legal, ceremonial, or religious dimensions of being married to each other. Gay and lesbian physicians are another large group of individuals who may present with their partners for couples therapy. They may or may not be married, have had a commitment ceremony, or have a domestic partnership agreement.

Common Complaints of Couples

What follows is a series of relationship symptoms and behaviors expressed by one or both members of a couple (see Table 10–1). Some of these constitute the "chief complaint" of medical couples, whereas others are uncovered in history taking. Some couples struggle with several concerns, and others may have only one or two complaints:

- *Trouble communicating.* "We don't talk enough"; "We can't talk about difficult issues"; "Our conversations are very superficial or boring."
- *Frequent arguments and fights.* "We can't seem to discuss things without a battle"; "We snipe at each other and nitpick about everything"; "We argue about the same things, over and over, there's no resolving of issues."
- *Violence.* "For the first time I hit my wife last weekend. I feel dreadful and ashamed—that's why I made this appointment for us"; "I'm in an abusive relationship; I want to separate; my husband needs individual help."
- *Sexual difficulties.* "We haven't made love in 9 months"; "We have sex, but it's not making love"; "I've developed erectile dysfunction."
- *Disagreements over the children.* "I'm tired of being the heavy-handed parent; my husband is Mr. Nice-Guy"; "My wife undermines my authority constantly—we're raising a couple of entitled, obnoxious brats."
- *Symptomatic child.* "Our son's been diagnosed with an autism spectrum disorder; we really need each other but his condition is driving a wedge between us."
- *Struggles with infertility.* "We've tried in vitro fertilization twice with no success. It's been very hard on our relationship, especially our communication and intimacy. We want some help before pursuing any other attempts of starting a family together."
- *Lack of time together.* "My wife is never home; pediatrics is very demanding"; "We only see each other on weekends, if that, given both of our careers."
- *Loneliness and isolation.* "I've gained 50 pounds since we moved here and my husband accepted this new job; I never see him; I graze on junk food."
- *Overwork and fatigue.* "I'm exhausted when I get home; I don't feel like talking"; "My husband is trying to build up his practice; he works 6 days a week, not much time for family."
- *Role strain in women physicians.* "My husband says that I hate sex; how frisky would you feel after practicing medicine full-time, raising three teenagers, chairing the hospital by-laws committee, looking in on your widowed father, singing in the church choir, and worrying about an abnormal mammogram?"
- *Fears or threats of divorce.* "My wife wants to leave, but I want to work on our relationship"; "We've both been married before—this is scary because neither of us wants to go through a divorce again."
- *Extramarital relationship.* "I've been having an affair for the past 6 months with another doctor at work. I just told my wife last week—we're here today to talk about next steps."
- *Dependencies on alcohol and other drugs.* "My partner has become an alcoholic—that's why we have no intimacy anymore"; "He's been off cocaine and marijuana now for over a year; we're here to begin to repair the marital erosion those drugs caused."

- *Psychiatric illness.* "I think my husband's got obsessive-compulsive disorder, but he argues that he's just a normal ophthalmologist—he's very controlling, and that's hard on me and the kids"; "I've been diagnosed with bipolar illness. It's been hard on my husband; our marriage has been severely tested with my two manic episodes."
- *Unemployed or underemployed spouse.* "I am so angry at my husband; he's lost his job and I have to return to my medical practice full time, not part-time, as soon as my maternity leave is up"; "I'm tired of being the breadwinner. Our kids are teenagers now and my wife refuses to return to nursing."
- *Coping with illness.* "My husband won't discuss his multiple sclerosis, and this is hard for me; we've become very distant from each other."
- *Intermarriage struggles.* "I am Korean and my husband is Jewish—surprise! Each of our families is not happy. Now we are pregnant and facing conflicts about baby naming and other rituals around his birth."
- *Unique issues for International Medical Graduates.* "We are fighting a lot. My husband is becoming very Westernized; he wants me to remove my hijab (headscarf), and he refuses to attend mosque with me. Even worse, I found porn sites bookmarked on his computer; this is disgusting. I want to leave America and return home."
- *Stepfamily issues.* "I've been married before; my wife hates my kids from that marriage, and they hate her."
- *Retirement challenges.* "I've given my husband an ultimatum—either he gives up his practice by the end of this year or I'm divorcing him"; "We bicker constantly; I'm worried about money, and my wife just ignores me. She says I've become depressed since I retired and that I need to see a psychiatrist."
- *Caring for elderly parents.* "I want my mother to come and live with us. She's had a mild stroke and needs assistance, but my husband says no"; "My father lives nearby and is a great help with our kids, but my wife resents him. She says he has no boundaries; he's around too much and touches her in a weird way sometimes. He's just lonely."

Impact of Addiction on the Couple

Addictive disorders (both chemical and nonchemical) are not uncommon in doctors and can have a profound impact on marital communication, emotional intimacy, and relationship stability and endurance (see Chapter 5, "Addictions: Chemical and Nonchemical"). However, addiction also occurs in the spouses and partners of physicians. Here is an example of addiction in the wife of a doctor:

TABLE 10–1. Frequent complaints of physicians and their spouses

- Poor communication
- Arguments and fights
- Physical/verbal abuse
- Sexual problems
- Issues with children
  - Conflicts over discipline
  - Problems in children
  - Infertility
- Lack of time together
  - Loneliness and isolation
  - Overwork and fatigue
- Role strain, especially in women
- Fear or threats of divorce
- Extramarital affairs
- Chemical dependency
- Psychiatric or physical illness in one member of couple
- Unemployed or underemployed spouse
- Cross-cultural issues
  - Intermarriage
  - Conflicts over religion or customs
- Retirement planning
- Care of elderly parents

Case Example

Dr. Ball was a 48-year-old family physician in a second marriage to Mrs. Ball, a 46-year-old retired flight attendant. They had been married for 15 years and had a 14-year-old daughter together. Dr. Ball had two daughters from his first marriage who lived several hundred miles away. He saw them at Christmas and in the summer for a couple of weeks. Mrs. Ball had a son from her first marriage who was married and living independently.

Dr. Ball began: "Why am I here? It's rather simple but a real mess. My wife's an alcoholic and in denial. I've tried everything and nothing works. She drinks every day. She's usually pretty gone when I get home from the office—or passed out. I don't keep any alcohol in the house. She drives to the liquor store and buys it. I've taken her keys away many times. She has it delivered. I find bottles hidden all over the house. We don't have friends anymore and haven't been to a party in years. She's embarrassing anyway. I think it's affecting Andrea, our daughter; they fight a lot and her grades have fallen. I don't like the kids she's hanging around with. She's out a lot in the evenings when I get home. I can't blame her. It's a rather depressing home. I make dinner but usually eat alone."

Dr. Ball continued: "I'm really worried about my wife's health. She hates doctors so I kind of treat her myself. I make sure she takes vitamins and folic acid. She has hypertension but I can't get her to take medication properly. She forgets, I guess, or is too drunk to care. I got her to take Antabuse for a while a few years ago. But she got really sick one day when she forgot that she took it and drank a fair bit of vodka. I also took her to Alcoholics Anonymous for a couple of visits. She felt that she didn't belong there. When she gets withdrawal symptoms, I give her Valium. And she gets a lot of headaches—real bad—but I don't give her narcotics. That's where I draw the line. But I worry about all of the Tylenol that she takes."

The psychiatrist completed a personal history on Dr. Ball and was not surprised to learn that he came from an alcoholic background. Both of his parents were heavy drinkers. In high school he had a part time job, helped with the bills when his parents were strapped, did a lot of work around the house, and looked after his younger brother. They were a "poor" family, and Dr. Ball was the first to go on to university. He got scholarships and worked all through college and medical school. He was married during internship. Regarding the demise of his first marriage, he told the psychiatrist that his wife got fed up with him, that he worked too hard, and she fell in love with another man.

The psychiatrist invited Mrs. Ball to come in for an interview but she refused. Couples therapy never took place. The psychiatrist reached out to Dr. Ball in four ways:

1. He suggested that Dr. Ball attend Alanon, which, after some initial reservation, he found very helpful.
2. He interviewed Andrea, their daughter. He found her to be a bright, psychologically sophisticated, but understandably angry young woman. She began attending Alateen and seeing a counselor at her school.
3. He recommended a local support group comprising male physicians whose wives had substance abuse problems. Dr. Ball benefited enormously from this safe, accepting, and largely upbeat gathering.
4. He helped Dr. Ball examine his experience while growing up, his tendency to "overdo" for others, his self-denial, his need to be needed, his tendency to be "enabling," and his problem with boundaries between being a husband and a physician to his wife. He insisted that his wife get her own primary care physician, and she did! At his last visit he said: "I feel a lot healthier now, and better equipped to make some decisions about my marriage."

This example illustrates some, but not all, of the ways in which addiction in a physician or his or her spouse affects marriage. See Table 10–2 for additional examples. Dr. Ball's story also demonstrates how a problem in the marriage sometimes must be managed by seeing only one member of the couple.

TABLE 10–2.   Effects of addiction on intimate relationships of physicians

- Denial, lying, and duplicity
- Vicious arguments while using, particularly when the drug of abuse is cocaine
- Physical violence and other forms of abuse (verbal, emotional, sexual)
- Avoidant behavior and/or icy silence
- Eroded intimacy
- Sexual dysfunction
- Sexual acting out
- Symptoms or symptomatic behavior in another or all family members (illustrative of the notion that addiction is a family disease)
- Financial strain
- Work impairment
- Boundary blurring, crossing, or violation
- Loss of health, respect, other relationships, status, and certainty

Love and the Medical Marriage

Spouses of physicians—and former spouses or partners of physicians—not uncommonly complain that their husband or wife has trouble with intimacy. When pressed, they describe a manner or style that is cool, detached, or intellectualized when trying to discuss deep or highly emotional matters. Some even describe a vocabulary that is devoid of tender, soft, or vulnerable language. They may go further and charge, usually erroneously, that the physician-partner is incapable of love or is stunted to some degree. Although some physicians do indeed have difficulty expressing or experiencing love, therapists of physicians also see those in the throes of love's ecstasy at one end of a continuum and physicians devastated by lost love at the other end.

Is it possible that medical study and the practice of medicine impair loving communication in medical marriages? As we noted in Chapter 1 ("The Psychology of Physicians and the Culture of Medicine"), the training of physicians gives ascendancy to science, rationalism, and intellectual defenses, including the liberal use of medical terminology and jargon. By omission and commission, the training of medical students and residents devalues emotion and the importance of love in the hearts of its students. The culture of medicine demands "objectivity" and "clinical neutrality" in its practitioners. Even empathy may be regarded as measured. In some physicians, this professional armor (which is adaptive and enables physicians to effectively perform their daily work) becomes hypertrophied and is sometimes carried from the workplace into the home. Giving and receiving love in the medical marriage becomes a challenge.

Case Example

Dr. Glen, a 44-year-old thoracic surgeon, consulted a psychiatrist about 4 weeks after his wife left him. He did not see it coming. She, on the other hand, argued that she had been trying to tell him for years that she was very unhappy, lonely, and bored in the marriage—he worked long hours and had a lot of medically related interests outside of his clinical work. She said that he never listened to her unhappy pleas for change or her wish to go with him for marital therapy. A few months before she left she met another man at work and started a relationship with him.

Dr. Glen was intensely mourning the loss of his wife. He told the psychiatrist about an incident that occurred in the operating room the previous week. Suddenly, he experienced a wave of sorrow come over him and his eyes filled with tears—a classical feature of grief when someone loses someone dear to them. When one of the nurses asked if he was okay, he replied: "Yes, I think I've developed some kind of allergy to this new disinfectant they're using here in the OR." It passed. When he was recounting this story in his psychiatrist's office, he said that he wished he could blurt out to the whole surgical team: "My eyes are like this because I can't stop crying—my wife is gone—my heart is broken!" Reflecting, Dr. Glen then said: "But how acceptable is that in the middle of a lung resection?"

Love in the medical marriage may also be masked by a host of character traits. In this case, the demands of sick patients and one doctor's "love" of his work blinded him to another kind of love—that of a spouse. This story also illustrates how tough it is to have a normal grief reaction and still do your job, especially if you are a male surgeon.

Complexity of a Presenting Complaint in Medical Marriages

Physicians can present with intricate challenges in their intimate relationships. Their stories fill the pages of DSM-IV-TR (American Psychiatric Association 2000b) and call for a thorough and broad-based assessment of etiological factors and an equally comprehensive and creative plan of treatment. Although couples therapy may be the treatment of choice and the only treatment necessary for some medical couples, many require attention paid to other illnesses or problems that are uncovered and that are outside the expertise or professional discipline of the couples therapist. It is not unusual that several health professionals are actively involved in the treatment of physicians (and their spouses and children) with complex comorbidity that has affected their health and relational life.

Case Examples: "We're Not Communicating"

Here are four snippets of medical couples, all with the same chief complaint of communication breakdown:

Case 1

Dr. Alexander and Mr. Blair have been married for 5 years and have 2 children. Dr. Alexander just finished her residency, and Mr. Blair just graduated from law school. They rarely get one-on-one time together. They have not made love in 6 months. They bicker constantly. Their nanny just quit. Assessment found nothing on Axis I, II, or III. The diagnosis is a V code—partner relational problem. They responded nicely to conjoint couples therapy.

Case 2

Dr. Martin and Dr. North, both psychiatrists, have been coupled for 6 years. Dr. Martin had a depression during his residency, but he has been off all medications for 2 years. Dr. North thinks that his partner is getting depressed again; he finds him irritable, withdrawn, emotionally flat, and sexually disinterested. He is also worried about his own mood; he has early morning awakening, teariness, unusual amounts of guilt, anhedonia, and forgetfulness. Assessment yielded major depressive disorder in each of them, and with treatment of the respective mood disorders their communication returned to normal.

Case 3

Dr. Castro had just been discharged from hospital after a manic episode. This was his third hospitalization in 2 years. Mrs. Castro is fed up with her husband's noncompliance with treatment, especially his medication. While manic he has had sex with prostitutes and spent a lot of money. She is very angry. Assessment of each of them found nothing of note in her case and an Axis I diagnosis of bipolar I disorder in her husband. Dr. Castro continued in treatment with his individual psychiatrist, and couples therapy was initiated by another psychiatrist. However, shortly into treatment, Dr. Castro stopped his medication yet again and became manic. While hospitalized involuntarily, his wife initiated divorce proceedings.

Case 4

Mrs. Dean was in the emergency department, having slashed her wrists after locking her husband out of the home for being drunk again. This was her third visit to emergency for cutting in 2 weeks. Dr. Dean is her fourth husband. She has three children, all of whom have been removed from her care because of neglect. Dr. Dean had been her psychiatrist, but he had stopped treatment and began a personal relationship with her. After 1 year, they married. She was his third wife. Last year he was diagnosed with prostate cancer and is undergoing treatment. Although Mrs. Dean has another psychiatrist, Dr. Dean still gives her pills when she runs out. On assessment, Mrs. Dean was given a diagnosis of borderline personality disorder. On Axis I, Dr. Dean was found to have alcohol dependence and rule out mood disorder due to a medical condition; on Axis II, a mixed personality disorder with narcissistic and dependent features; on Axis III, prostate cancer. Dr. Dean was suspended from practicing medicine and attended residential treatment for his alcoholism. While he was there, Mrs. Dean began a relationship with someone else, but she ended it when her husband returned. Couples therapy only lasted three visits. Dr. Dean stated that he could not regain his trust for her and moved out of their home.

With the exception of Case 1, it is clear how much having an illness affects communication. The therapeutic imperative is to treat any illness on Axis I or III at the same time as—or instead of—beginning couples treatment. Often Axis II disorders must be addressed in individual therapy as well, in combination with couples work.

Couples Therapy With Physicians: Basic Principles

There is no unitary approach to distressed medical couples that present for couples therapy. The marriage and family therapy literature does not identify physicians as having particularly unique relationships that warrant specialized study or research. Hence, trained therapists probably apply general principles to their therapy with physician couples, albeit with their individual and subjective style. Here is one such approach.

The first visit is usually a conjoint one—that is, both the physician and his or her spouse or partner come together and are invited to articulate and express their respective "chief complaint(s)." Their concerns may be the same or different. Both are asked to discuss their feelings about the other's concerns. Exposition of their problems and the associated emotions may consume most of the time allotted for the initial visit. By the end of that visit, the therapist should have a great deal of information about what they consider their "problem list." Issues raised toward the end of the visit will need elaboration at a later point. The therapist may also learn about the duration of symptoms (and whether they agree or disagree on the timeline) and their impact on each of the partners. How demoralized is each of them? How do they feel about the viability of their relationship? Have they sought couples therapy in the past, and if so, how was that for each of them?

The therapist should preserve some time to ask about the strengths of the relationship and the ways in which they still function as a healthy couple. Individuals appreciate this line of questioning, and even if they are struggling to find positive aspects of their relationship, they will welcome any affirming and spontaneous feedback, no matter how small, from the therapist. Examples might include "I agree that your problems are serious and divisive, and your being here together today says that you care enough about each other—and your children—to face this together, and with a complete stranger. That's never easy" or "The difficulties that you two are having are common ones that I see in dual-doctor marriages. It's good that you've come now rather than later. I feel confident that I can help."

Before stopping, the therapist should try to give a brief summary of what he or she thinks are the main problems and challenges, present a general and tentative treatment plan, and invite questions and comments from each of them. This last point is key because it communicates that the work will be collaborative—that the therapist will be helping them to help themselves as they work on their marriage. Medical couples often express concern about confidentiality: what information is shared and with whom? Who has access to any written notes? Is a consultation dictated and sent to a referring person? Is this covered by insurance? What options exist to pay privately?

The next two visits are 1-hour sessions with each person alone. The therapist conducts a detailed assessment with particular emphasis on developmental dynamics both in the family and personal histories. Each person is told that the visits are for the therapist's purposes, to gain important knowledge about each of them and the ways in which they complement each other and the ways in which they clash. They should be reassured that information from the individual visits will not be brought into future conjoint meetings (with the exception of material that they have obviously shared with each other and is not a secret to the other). Gaining each individual's trust enables the partners to disclose to the therapist information that they have never revealed to the spouse but that represents fragments of a life that they want the therapist to know about. Examples might include a therapeutic abortion while in college, a homosexual experience during medical or graduate school, a previous and annulled marriage, being the victim of sexual abuse by an older sibling, or a previous depression and suicide attempt at an earlier time in life. The therapist must decide with each person what is relevant to their current relationship difficulties and what is not. It is possible that some individual therapy will be deemed necessary.

The individual visits also give the therapist an opportunity to do a DSM-IV-TR multiaxial assessment. As in the previous section, it is important to rule in or out any diagnoses on Axis I, II, and III. Some individuals presenting for couples therapy will already be in the midst of treatment with someone else for a diagnosis that has been made earlier. Others will not be, and it will be necessary for the couples therapist to ensure that a referral is made to someone else to treat, for example, a suspected mood disorder, cannabis abuse, or posttraumatic stress disorder. Some psychiatrists, especially in smaller or remote communities with scant mental health resources, will shift gears and forgo couples treatment while they treat the individual(s) on a one-on-one basis for whatever the psychiatric disorder is. They may or may not resume couples therapy later, depending upon its necessity, passage of time, and the wishes of each of the partners.

In most couples therapy formats, visit number four and subsequent visits are conjoint in nature. The gravity of the problems, their duration and urgency, and how well the partners are able to function both as individuals and as a couple will in large measure dictate the type of psychotherapy. Couples in high distress who are overwhelmed, regressed, and on the verge of separating require a supportive approach. Couples in conflict but with moderate resilience respond well to interpretative therapy and interventional strategies. Seasoned therapists who have treated many physician couples remark on the value of an eclectic approach encompassing psychodynamic, systems, cognitive-behavioral, interpersonal, and relational theories and strategies (Miller and Stiver 1997).

The basic themes of relational theory make it particularly applicable to the couples treatment of physicians (Bergman and Surrey 2004). It recognizes the powerful impact of intrapsychic factors, particularly internal object relations, and cultural context on the lives of women and men. Relationships are seen as the central organizing feature in people's development. There is an appreciation of women's and men's relational patterns. Problems are addressed, but potential strengths are also emphasized as providing a new pathway for healthy growth and development. Women and men search to connect with others.

Other therapists, especially psychiatrists, include biological considerations in their approach to medical couples—a mindfulness about how untreated or undertreated Axis I disorders affect marital communication, how medications affect a couple's sexual interest and functioning, how street drugs can cause mood lability and irritability in the relationship dyad, and how frontal lobe disease can cause disinhibition and inappropriate behavior that embarrasses the spouse. Given the ethnic and racial diversity of today's medical couples, it is essential that all couples therapists strive to practice culturally competent treatment (Lim 2006). It is acceptable, if not desirable, to ask couples whose ethnicity or race are different than one's own about norms and values of their respective culture. Similarly, when treating couples who are intermarried, therapists must watch for alignments and clashes with their own reference group if one member of the couple is of the same race, ethnicity, or faith.

Gender is another important variable in couples therapy with physicians. All therapists must consider how their being a man or a woman influences how they are perceived by one or both partners in the relationship. As with culture and race, one must watch for same-gender and cross-gender identifications and dissonance when treating couples. There are occasions when it is therapeutic and rapport-building to be quite explicit about this. Couples who are struggling with role conflict in the home (especially division of household labor), including sexist attitudes in one or both of them, appreciate being able to talk openly with a therapist who is the same gender as one of them and the opposite gender of the other. The capacity to be as neutral as one can be and to empathize with each of them is fundamental in situations such as these.

When treating medical couples in which one is a physician and the other is not, the therapist must be especially sensitive to this fact. The nonmedical spouse may fear an automatic alliance between his or her spouse and the treating psychiatrist. Likewise, the psychiatrist must be wary of not identifying or counter-identifying more with the physician spouse than the nonphysician partner. Two problems are most common and point to this kind of error. First is enabling—that is, the treating psychiatrist normalizes overwork in the physician spouse and the ascendancy of medical practice over the responsibilities of marriage and family. Second is "ganging up" on the physician spouse by colluding with the nonmedical spouse.

When treating dual-physician marriages, the psychiatrist should consider countertransference "blind spots." Asking oneself questions may be helpful: Would a nonmedical therapist—a psychologist or clinical social worker—assess this couple differently than me? Is my understanding of each of them and my focus biologically skewed? Are antidepressants or other medications really necessary? Am I using too much medical jargon and terminology with them? Am I reinforcing their use of intellectualization as a defense? Are we really dealing with underlying dynamic issues? There may not be alignment or clashing around profession (because we are all physicians), but what about gender and specialty? Do I show favoritism to the psychiatrist spouse in a psychiatrist–surgeon marriage? Are my own psychological vulnerabilities activated by either partner? Am I repeating something from my own past here? Are the conflicts in this marriage too close to those in my own?

Being flexible in one's approach is key. In some couples, individual therapy for one or both of the partners will be necessary. In some situations, individual treatment proceeds simultaneously with the conjoint work. In others, it may be sequential; that is, the conjoint work ceases temporarily or indefinitely while one or both receive(s) individual care. Couples therapists need to understand that conjoint work can be more intimidating for patients than individual treatment. The major reason for this is that patients have more control in individual therapy. They can titrate how much they disclose to their therapist depending upon their level of trust, readiness, pace, and so forth. In conjoint treatment, either partner fears being blindsided, confronted, or shamed by their spouse who brings up an issue for discussion that he or she is not ready to face.

Benefits of Couples Therapy

There are several ways in which couples therapy can be helpful for medical marriages. Individuals in the midst of marital conflict and unhappiness, including physicians and their spouses, can have enormous difficulty identifying relationship issues. Even with some insight by one or both of them in delineating core areas of discord or dissonance, they may be blind to predisposing, precipitating, and perpetuating factors unique to their relationship. Furthermore, they may erroneously or naively attribute causation to one or more surface stressors without appreciating the power of long-standing intrapsychic and interpersonal dynamics. A common example is blaming the physician's long hours at the hospital for blighted communication. Overwork may be part of it, but sometimes it is the other way around—that is, there is a fundamental difficulty with intimate communication in one or both of them. Stalemates and thwarted attempts at intimate talking abound. The physician spends increasing amounts of time at work to avoid dealing with unresolved marital matters.

In a survey of 134 physicians and 125 physician spouses (Gabbard et al. 1987), the physicians rated the amount of time away from home at work as a much more important source of conflict than the spouses did. The spouses, on the other hand, considered lack of intimacy a much more serious problem than the physicians did. The investigators concluded that the lack of time due to the demands of practice seems to be a complaint physicians use to externalize the conflicts in the marriage regarding intimacy and communication onto factors *outside* the marriage. In this regard, the excessive time demands that characterize the lives of most physicians may be more of a *symptom* of the marital problems than the *cause*. Physicians may need to stay away from home. They may prefer the office, where their lives are structured and they have more of a sense of mastery and control, over their home lives, where things are spontaneous and not within their control (see Chapter 1). As this research suggests, both members of a couple may be convinced that the time demands of the culture of medicine are at the root of the difficulties. One way that couples therapy can be extremely helpful is to clarify the underlying problems of emotional connection that are at the core of the conflicts within the couple. As one spouse of a physician said in a marital session, "Even when he is home, he's not really there."

Another benefit of couples therapy is that each of the partners feels heard and validated by the therapist. Both are usually starving for this experience because they are not able to receive these basic needs from each other or give back. In fact, it may be worse; not only do they feel unsupported by the other but they also feel diminished or confused. The alliance of couplehood that characterizes functional and healthy relationships is lacking, and each may be struggling with faltering self-confidence and wobbly self-esteem. In addition to identifying and clarifying issues that need therapeutic work, the therapist is also a facilitator of the couple's communication. He or she can ease the exposition of tough and conflict-laden subjects in the therapy sessions, giving relief to the individuals. With time and encouragement, this enables them to continue these types of conversations at home.

Depending upon the specifics of the medical couple, the therapist can invite and modulate affect in each of the partners. By paraphrasing and modeling more effective ways of saying what needs to be said, the therapist helps spouses who feel intimidated or shut down by the intense affect of their husband or wife. This contrasts with the situation in which a spouse is completely frustrated by or avoidant of the husband or wife who speaks with minimal to no affect; the therapist cuts through the intellectualized language and tone to release feelings. In simple terms, the therapist creates a safe place for the two individuals to speak frankly and intimately with each other.

Yet another benefit of couples therapy is that a therapist can outline the architecture of the impasse between the couple. Each partner generally approaches couples therapy with the assumption (and hope) that the therapist will see the problem as residing in the other spouse or partner and facilitate that spouse or partner's change. In fact, they will learn that conflicts in a relationship are almost always two-way and that negotiation and compromise are the keys to getting out of the impasse. Each must acknowledge his or her own contributions and try to meet the other halfway in modifying the interactions in the relationship. Moreover, couples therapy may provide tools for communicating that the partners previously lacked (Jones and Gabbard 1988). A good couples therapist helps the members of the couple learn to talk from the "I" perspective rather than to simply blame or accuse the partner. They may learn not to negotiate by ultimatum, in which one threatens the other. They also can be taught to make their needs explicit rather than to expect the spouse or partner to rely on mind reading. Fundamentally they will learn that change is primarily the responsibility of both members of the couple and that the therapist cannot change either one of them.

Couples therapy may also uncover unconscious contracts that were tacitly forged at the time the relationship began (Jones and Gabbard 1988). A wife, for example, may unconsciously expect her husband to act like a dependent child so she can pamper him, and the husband may unconsciously expect his wife to mother him. These expectations may never be spoken but are enacted continuously. When genograms are done for both partners, the evolution of these patterns may be clearly related to transgenerational themes in the families of origin.

In cases where the physician member of the couple may have problems with mentalization, as described in Chapter 6 ("Personality Disorders, Personality Traits, and Disruptive Physicians"), couples therapy may offer a benefit beyond what individual therapy provides. The physician with narcissistic personality disorder, for example, may have a great deal of difficulty understanding why he is mired in recurrent problems with colleagues in the workplace. The recommendation of individual therapy may not be welcomed because the physician is not really convinced that he or she has problems that warrant individual therapy. On the other hand, when the spouse is included in the couples therapy process, the spouse may be able to serve as a loving and supportive source of feedback on how the physician comes across to others.

Case Example

Dr. Martin and his wife came to evaluation because Dr. Martin had had numerous complaints made about him in the hospital, especially from nursing staff. He worked in neonatal intensive care, and he repeatedly berated nurses whom he felt were not doing their job in taking care of very ill infants. He was on the verge of being suspended from the medical staff, and he was convinced that there was a conspiracy against him in the hospital. He maintained that his goal was to provide excellent care and that he was not appreciated.

His wife willingly entered couples therapy with him as a way of helping him see what he could not see himself. She would say to him in the couples therapy, "You have to be right all the time, honey. You have the best intentions in the world, but you make others feel like their opinions don't matter. In fact, if others have good ideas, you can't accept them because you didn't think of them first."

As the couple's therapy proceeded, Dr. Martin would bring instances from the workplace into the treatment, and Mrs. Martin would help him see why nurses might feel the way they do when he interacts with them in a way that feels demeaning to them. She said that she herself often felt dismissed by him, and she suggested to him that his abruptness might cause nurses in the neonatal intensive care to feel similarly dismissed.

In this manner, the couples therapy served almost as an assisted individual therapy in which the doctor's wife was functioning as a mirror held up to the physician to help him see how others see him. This approach allowed Dr. Martin to become more reflective about himself and increase his capacity to mentalize the experience of others. This example also illustrates another benefit of couples therapy. The spouse may be of enormous help in gently confronting the physician with his grandiose view of himself. A loving spouse reminds the physician that he puts his trousers on in the morning like everyone else. In other words, the spouse should not take the idealization expressed by the physician's patients seriously.

Discouragement about a future together is quite common in medical couples requesting help with their marriage. In part, this is because they have procrastinated and delayed seeking assistance; in other words, the problems are longstanding and entrenched. However, many discouraged couples actually have a viable relationship, but it is impossible for them to see that or to feel hopeful. Some married physicians have had a huge and inordinate number of changes or stressors in a relatively short period of time. It is akin to "system overload," with each party working very hard simply to survive. Each may feel very alone, unsupported, and cynical about their marital foundation.

Case Example

A psychiatrist received a telephone call that began like this: "This is Mark Abrams calling. I don't know if you remember me or not, but you helped me during my residency when my wife and I split up. Well I'm in trouble again. My wife—I got married again 5 years ago—has asked me to move out. Can you see us?"

In the first visit with Dr. Abrams and his wife, Dr. Wong, here is what came out:

- Dr. Wong had also been married before and divorced during her residency. She met Dr. Abrams when they were both completing fellowships in gynecological oncology.
- After dating for 9 months, they got married and started a family right away. They had two daughters ages 4 years and 9 months, respectively.
- They worked at the same medical center; Dr. Abrams worked "more than full time" (according to Dr. Wong), and Dr. Wong worked "much more than her so-called part time" (according to Dr. Abrams). There were professional stressors—unhappiness with their new department head, a merger, worries about their salaries and research grants, and concerns about academic progression.
- They were extremely tense together, interrupted each other repeatedly, were both very guarded, competed constantly to get the psychiatrist's attention, and sat as far apart on the couch as they possibly could. They seemed exhausted and demoralized.

The psychiatrist summed up their first visit trying to be as upbeat as possible. He pointed out that they had had phenomenal changes in their lives: completion of decades of education and specialty training, passing board examinations, landing their first "jobs," a major geographical relocation for each, a relatively brief courtship, a very short period of marriage without kids, and now two young children—all of this in only 5 years! Because they had each been married before, the psychiatrist wondered aloud if they might be anxious about this relationship floundering and worried that they might divorce again.

They both nodded in response, and in unison said to the other: "Oh, my god, I didn't know you felt like this too." Dr. Abrams then turned to the psychiatrist: "I think I've got tons of baggage, with my mom and dad splitting up when I was a teenager and my own marriage going down the tubes when I was a resident, I don't have a hell of a lot of confidence in my ability to really make a marriage survive." Dr. Wong said, "I give myself straight A's studying, doing research, and teaching, but when it comes to my personal life, I don't know myself and what I want or need."

The psychiatrist explained how he worked, presented a plan for the next few visits, and invited and answered questions. As the session ended and everyone stood up, he said to them: "Perhaps we will also discuss what it's like for you two to be in an intermarriage, how it's been for your folks, your kids, and so forth." They both laughed and shook their heads wearily. Dr. Abrams said: "Wait till you hear our stories. We're right up there with the heartache of the Middle East and Northern Ireland." Dr. Wong smiled warmly at him and reached for his hand as they left the office.

Follow-up visits totaled six in all. In those sessions, Drs. Abrams and Wong talked openly with each other about feeling interrupted and misunderstood. They discussed the fatigue that each of them felt. They needed to renegotiate division of labor in the home; Dr. Wong was clearly doing more than her share, and once Dr. Abrams could see that, he was happy to pitch in more. They discussed ways in which they could each get a bit more alone time, and they found a way to protect time for each other for "dates." They spoke about a common sorrow—and loss—that each of their respective families was not accepting of their marriage. This gave them some measure of solidarity, but it was bittersweet. When they stopped treatment they were feeling much better as individuals and as a couple.

Not all demoralized couples have such a happy ending. When the medical marriage is dead, toxic, or on life support, couples therapy can be very helpful in affirming that state of paralysis or heartache. Should the couple decide to separate, the therapist can assist them with the details of this and the many emotions associated with impending separation—sadness, relief, anger, guilt and failure, anxiety, and more. Not uncommonly, the partners will be at different points of bereavement; that is, despite the appearance of mutuality in the agreement to live apart, one is usually hurting more than the other. One may also be more bitter than the other or holding on more tenaciously. The therapist, as an advocate for each of them, can point this out to enhance the other's empathy and patience during this difficult transition. The therapeutic imperative is to help them separate with less pain and rancor and with more dignity. Discussions about the potential and actual impact of separation on children are crucial and always welcomed by each party. Some therapists will hold at least one session with the children, when age appropriate, for questions and guidance and referral to a child or adolescent mental health professional if indicated.

Conclusion

Couples therapy is a significant modality of treatment for all people in a troubled relationship, but there is at least one reason why it is important in married physicians, especially those who are clinicians and in caretaking roles: People feel more capable of caring when they are cared for, more able to give when they feel happy, and more inclusive when they feel loved and appreciated. The message for physicians is obvious: "You cannot fully help your patients if you do not take care of yourselves and your families and receive care in return from them." Physicians who have been helped by couples therapy can attest to its power outside the home. They now approach their work with greater vitality and renewed vigor.

Key Points

- Physicians not uncommonly have problems in their marriages and can benefit from couples therapy.

- For a host of reasons—stigma, denial, busyness, pride, rugged individualism (especially in male physicians), contempt for therapy, and more—physicians tend to delay seeking much-needed marital help.

- The marital conflicts of physicians are not unlike those of other busy professionals, but their embarrassment about them and their reluctance to seek help mean that significant erosion of function and intimacy may have occurred by the time of the initial consultation.

- Because physicians are prone to depression and substance abuse and dependence (or both), their marriages may be severely compromised by these illnesses.

- Couples therapy with physicians requires an eclectic approach, grounded in biopsychosocial principles, so that the relationship and each of its players are well served.

- Given the cultural pluralism of today's physicians, couples therapy must be sensitive to how marital and family values both inform and clash with contemporary medical practice.

The Suicidal Physician and the Aftermath of Physician Suicide

> No one who has not been there can comprehend the suffering leading up to suicide, nor can they really understand the suffering of those left behind in the wake of suicide.
>
> Kay Redfield Jamison (2006)

We began this book with a notation of the tragic death by suicide of Dr. Jonathan Drummond-Webb, chief of pediatric and congenital cardiac surgery at the Arkansas Children's Hospital in Little Rock, Arkansas (see Chapter 1, "The Psychology of Physicians and the Culture of Medicine"). Our intent was to examine the life and death of Dr. Drummond-Webb in order to illustrate the psychology of physicians—especially their personalities—that in part explains their psychiatric morbidity. In this chapter, we discuss what is known about the epidemiology, risk factors, assessment, and treatment of suicidal physicians. Suicide prevention is central and pivotal in decreasing the numbers of doctors who kill themselves each year, so we outline preventive strategies. We also describe the impact of physician suicide on family members, friends, medical colleagues, and patients.

Epidemiology

Schernhammer and Colditz's (2004) review and meta-analysis of 25 studies on physician suicide concluded that the aggregate suicide rate ratio for male physicians, compared with the general population, is 1.41:1. For female physicians, the ratio is 2.27:1. According to the American Foundation for Suicide Prevention (2002), studies in the past 40 years have confirmed that physicians die by suicide more frequently than others of their gender and age both in the general population and in other professional occupations. On average, death by suicide is about 70% more likely among male physicians in the United States than among other professionals, and 250%–400% higher among female physicians. Unlike almost all other population groups, in which men die by suicide about four times more frequently than women, physicians have a suicide rate that is very similar for both men and women. The American Foundation for Suicide Prevention formed a work group, whose members argued, in their published consensus statement (Center et al. 2003), that the culture of medicine accords low priority to physician mental health despite evidence of untreated mood disorders and an increased burden of suicide. The work group recommended transforming professional attitudes and changing institutional policies to encourage physicians to seek help.

Are there differences in rates of suicide by physicians in various branches of medicine? Hawton et al. (2001), employing a retrospective cohort study of physicians in England and Wales who died by suicide between 1979 and 1995, found that there were significant differences between specialties, with anesthesiologists, community health doctors, general practitioners, and psychiatrists having significantly increased rates compared with doctors in general hospital medicine. Regarding methods, their study found that self-poisoning with drugs was more common among doctors (including those who were retired) than in general-population suicides (Hawton et al. 2000). Barbiturates were the most frequent drugs used. Half of the anesthesiologists who died used anesthetic agents. Self-cutting was also more frequently used as a method of suicide. To our knowledge there are no physician suicide studies that are more current or that track the specialty or the means of suicide in North American doctors.

Why Do Physicians Kill Themselves?

As we noted in Chapter 1, the act of suicide is a complex phenomenon involving some convergence of genes, psychology, and psychosocial stressors. Suicide experts believe that 85%–90% of individuals who die by suicide have been living with some type of psychiatric illness, whether diagnosed or not. Despite the basic medical knowledge that all physicians possess about psychiatric disorders, es-

TABLE 11–1. Profile of a physician at high risk for suicide

Gender	Male or female
Age	45+ years old if female; 50+ years old if male
Race	White
Marital status	Divorced, separated, single, or currently with marital disruption
Habits	Alcohol or other drug abuse "Workaholic" Excessive risk taker (especially high-stakes gambler; thrill seeker)
Medical status	Psychiatric symptoms (especially depression; anxiety) Physical symptoms (chronic pain; chronic debilitating illness)
Professional	Change in status: threat to status, autonomy, security, financial stability, recent losses, increased work demands
Access to means	Access to lethal medications Access to firearms

Source. Reprinted from Silverman MM: "Physicians and Suicide," in *The Handbook of Physician Health.* Edited by Goldman LS, Myers M, Dickstein LJ. Chicago, IL, American Medical Association, 2000. Copyright 2000, American Medical Association. Used with permission.

pecially depression, and the availability of medical care for them, an unknown number of physicians kill themselves each year who "fall through the cracks." These are physicians who have never been assessed by a mental health professional or been given any form of treatment. They may or may not have tried to treat themselves.

Silverman (2000), in a significant review of published research, concluded that there are additional factors that put physicians at risk of suicide (see Table 11–1). Considering diagnostic nosology, the author found that the psychiatric disorders in Table 11–2 are the ones most commonly associated with physician suicide.

An addendum to Silverman's at-risk factor and diagnostic grouping is in order. First, dual diagnoses are very common in physicians, especially the dangerous combination of substance abuse or dependence and mood disorders. However, comorbid conditions of substance disorders and anxiety disorders, eating disorders, and dementia can also put physicians at risk for suicidal behavior. Second, we have no current data on suicide risk or rates in medical students, residents, minority physicians (ethnic, racial, religious, gay, lesbian, transgendered), or International Medical Graduates. This type of information is critical and

TABLE 11–2.   Psychiatric disorders associated with physician suicide

- Major depressive disorder

- Bipolar affective disorder

- Alcohol and other drug abuse

- Anxiety disorders, including panic disorder

- Borderline personality disorder

Source.   Reprinted from Silverman MM: "Physicians and Suicide," in *The Handbook of Physician Health.* Edited by Goldman LS, Myers M, Dickstein LJ. Chicago, IL, American Medical Association, 2000. Copyright 2000, American Medical Association. Used with permission.

would be very helpful in knowing what groups within medicine might be more vulnerable than others and could benefit from prevention strategies.

In addition to demographic and diagnostic factors that may put a physician at risk for self-harm, other specifics are important. Table 11–3 lists some considerations in history-taking that contribute to a more comprehensive suicide risk assessment in the ill physician.

The stress-diathesis model (Mann et al. 1999) is helpful in trying to understand why physicians kill themselves. The risk for suicidal acts is determined not solely by the presence of a psychiatric illness (the stressor) but also by a diathesis. This diathesis, which is present in some but not all patients, includes a tendency to experience more suicidal ideation and a tendency toward impulsivity, especially in the face of overwhelming stress. What results is a heightened likelihood of acting on suicidal feelings.

Case Example

Dr. Gregory, a third-year resident in surgery, came to see a psychiatrist about 6 weeks after slipping into a clinical depression. He described his mood as flat and dull. He had lost about 7 pounds of weight; he was having some difficulty concentrating and was awakening early in the morning; and his self-confidence was down. He was not suicidal. Because he had had a similar episode in medical school (and had been treated by the same psychiatrist), he knew what was wrong with him. He was prescribed the same antidepressant he had taken before and was scheduled to return in a week. The evening before that follow-up visit the psychiatrist received a phone call from Dr. Gregory's partner, Dr. Rand, who was a resident in psychiatry. He was in a panic and told the psychiatrist that Dr. Gregory was acutely suicidal. Dr. Rand had come home from work to find him standing out on the balcony of their twenty-first-floor apartment and debating whether to jump. It was in the middle of winter. Dr. Rand grabbed onto him and pulled him back inside. "It was like he was in a dissociative state, very weird, kind of

TABLE 11–3. Suicide risk considerations in physicians

- *Previous history of a depressive episode*—this may have occurred in adolescence or young adulthood, college, or medical school, and whether recognized and treated or not, this is significant information.

- *Previous suicide attempt*—physician deaths by suicide are distinct from the general public because of the relative paucity of previous suicide attempts. However, some physicians have attempted suicide before and survived. Most feel deeply embarrassed and will not disclose this matter easily to their treating physician.

- *Family history of mood disorders, including suicide*—many physicians have genetic loading for mood disorders. Suicide can be familial, but it is much more complicated than genetic predisposition.

- *Professional isolation*—this may be longstanding in someone who tends to be a loner, very private, and/or self-contained. More commonly, professional isolation is the result of a geographic move or loss of some type (health, family, financial stability). These individuals lack the supports and the protective factors that militate against self-destruction (American Psychiatric Association 2004).

- *Lawsuits and medical license investigations*—being sued for malpractice or having complaints made to one's licensing board about professional competence, safety, or ethics can be one of the most traumatic assaults to a physician's health and sense of well-being. Such individuals, especially if alone without actual or perceived supports, are at risk of self-harm.

- *Poor treatment adherence*—for whatever reason—denial, shame, simple ignorance—some physicians are not very good patients. They cannot accept the gravity of their illness(es) and the pressing need for professional help (Jamison 1999). Their symptoms worsen and they lose hope. If they have an associated unchecked substance abuse problem, they are especially at risk of killing themselves.

- *Treatment-refractory psychiatric illness*—like patients in general, some physicians have "malignant" psychiatric disorders that do not respond easily to state-of-the-art psychiatric treatment. When one is symptomatic for long periods of time or achieves very short (or increasingly short) periods of remission, demoralization sets in and suicide risk builds.

dazed. Once I sat him down inside and just held onto him, he came around and just started sobbing. I was terrified, but very relieved at the same time," said Dr. Rand.

It was fortuitous that the psychiatrist was actually on call and at the hospital seeing patients with his resident. Drs. Gregory and Rand lived nearby, so, assured that Dr. Gregory was indeed safe now, he made a house call. He learned that that afternoon, Dr. Gregory had been grilled and berated by his attending physician at the bedside of a postoperative patient for not being up-to-date regarding the patient's condition. He had been up all night on call. He had been humiliated in front of the other residents and medical students also at the bedside. In fact, the patient had said to the attending physician: "Forgive me for butting in sir, but aren't you being a little hard on my doctor?" Later, upon arriving home from work, Dr. Gregory mused: "I think that my attending physician is right—I really am a loser. I think they made a mistake letting me into this residency. I'm just taking up space here." He began to think that he was better off dead. He said, "So, I opened the sliding door to the balcony, just to look down, just to see if jumping might work. I was only out there a few minutes I think when Bill got home." The psychiatrist arranged for a brief inpatient stay until the suicidal crisis had passed and Dr. Gregory's mood began improving.

What this example illustrates is the progression to suicidal behavior and an aborted and lethal suicide attempt. The suicidal diathesis was provoked by a humiliating stressor at work (or narcissistic injury) on top of a recurrent mood disorder, partially treated, which was probably aggravated by sleep deprivation and fatigue as immediate and proximal factors. This man experienced other emotions at the bedside besides embarrassment—he also felt anxious and agitated—and this made him impulsive and at high risk of hurting himself. There is a pressing imperative in this story—that what is normative in some residency programs (aggressive and shaming teaching, sleep loss, and tiredness) can be dangerous and life threatening when a trainee's resilience is broken by illness.

Another caveat is in order. A physician does not have to have depression to become lethally suicidal when a narcissistic injury is inflicted. Although much is made of mood disorders and alcoholism in the suicide literature, narcissistic vulnerability is given far less emphasis. A diagnosis of narcissistic personality disorder is not necessary to have a fragile self-esteem that is easily wounded. Perfectionistic physicians are likely to feel that any error in judgment is a sign of failure or incompetence and thus overreact. Those blows to self-esteem that are damaging to one's public reputation—such as a lawsuit or an investigation for Medicare fraud—may be especially powerful. We know of several cases in which suicide or a serious attempt followed such narcissistic insults almost immediately, long before depression had time to take hold. For some physicians the loss of face is so unbearable that suicide seems the only way out.

A word about stigma is also in order. Many physicians, especially when living with a psychiatric illness, have heightened internalized stigma. They feel deeply ashamed, diminished, and tend to pull away from others. This increases an inner sense of aloneness that may already be present as a symptom of their mood or anxiety disorder. Melancholia, guilt, and cognitive distortion are common symptoms of depression; these symptoms may be worsened in physicians who tend to be perfectionistic and self-castigating anyway. Internalized stigma rests within the physician him- or herself. However, there is also cultural stigma, a stigma that resides within the house of medicine. Judgmental, ignorant, and discriminatory attitudes toward physicians living with mental illness compound their suffering, increase isolation, foster an "us and them" mentality, delay help-seeking, reinforce denial of illness, drive self-treatment, and heighten the risk of suicide in doctors. Changing this stigma is one of the greatest challenges for our profession in the twenty-first century. Its eradication will not only lower the number of physicians who die by suicide each year but also ensure that ill physicians get much needed treatment earlier.

What Can We Learn From Physicians Who Have Attempted Suicide But Did Not Die?

A recently published first-person account (quoted in Myers and Fine 2006) is both chilling and illuminating:

> I lost complete consciousness the moment I jumped—I was jumping into oblivion. I was in the intensive care unit for almost 2 months;—it took me one month to regain consciousness. I had no recollection of what happened. I remember asking, "Did I commit suicide?"
>
> This happened 3 years ago when I was in my first year of medical residency. I was beginning to feel overwhelmed and became consumed with feelings of worthlessness and inadequacy. I started to think about suicide all the time. I didn't have a concrete plan to kill myself; my feelings of wanting to die were more passive like wishing that I would disappear or no longer exist. I read a story about an elderly woman who had been hit by a bus and died instantly, and I remember feeling guilty about wanting that for myself. I also had thoughts of a knife stabbing me, although I never went to the drawer and looked at the knives.
>
> One morning, a short while after I had returned from being on call overnight, I was in my apartment and realized that I did have a way out—I could jump off my balcony. I started telling myself that I wasn't meant for this life, that the world would be better without me. The rational part of me was not working—I would have never chosen such a public death as jumping into the street. At that moment it did not occur to me that I might be unsuccessful at dying.
>
> I went to the ledge of the balcony at least two times, looked down, then returned to the couch. I was very ambivalent, and then suddenly the telephone rang and it was my program director. I couldn't disguise the fact that I was crying and what I was contemplating. He asked for my address, saying that he would send the chief resident over immediately.
>
> I had this thought that I was insulted. How could my director send over a complete stranger and not come himself? I had just confided something so intimate, so personal to another human being, and I did not expect the response that I got. Suddenly, my ambivalence became a resolution. I didn't want anyone

to think what I was doing was manipulation. I told my program director that this is something I have to do and jumped off the balcony.

I thought it was cruel that I was allowed to survive. My apartment was on the sixth floor—I should have realized that there was a chance I wouldn't die. My injuries included pulmonary hemorrhages, rib fractures, ruptured spleen, abdominal hemorrhages, fractured jaw, a fractured wrist, fractured vertebrae, and a spinal cord transection at T4, which means that I'm paralyzed from the chest down.

My future? I am now planning to return to residency, but the specifics will depend on further assessment of my psychological abilities. I still have feelings of hopelessness and worthlessness, but I'm looking forward to practicing medicine again. I have always had a feeling of warmth and love for humanity and see medicine as a way for me to express that love.

When I was in the rehabilitation center, one of my psychiatrists, who had known me during medical school, told me "You do belong in medicine." His faith in me had a very powerful effect—he said this to me when I was being so hard on myself. But he believed in me, and now I also will try to believe in myself.

Dr. Khadilkar's courage in sharing this very private story is a gift to others, especially his medical colleagues. Very few physicians speak so openly about their mental illness, let alone suicidal actions. There are lessons in his narrative: that physicians are no different than the general public and are subject to psychiatric illnesses; that some physicians descend into depression but keep working, perhaps trying to be strong and hoping that by serving others their symptoms may go away; that passive suicidal ideation is not rare in physicians, especially trainees; that when a physician is post-call, he or she may be more vulnerable to suicidal acts; that there is ambivalence about dying in most suicidal people; and that even after traumatic injury from a suicide attempt a physician may return to (and be welcomed back into) medical training and practice.

Most important is that Dr. Khadilkar has chipped away at stigma in the world of medicine by speaking so candidly. Spritz (quoted in Myers and Fine 2006), Pare (2006), and Baxter (1998) are some other physicians who have written first-person accounts of their psychiatric illnesses and suicide attempts. All three physicians chronicle their anguish and desperation, salute the excellent psychiatric care they received, and, grateful to be alive, bring a palpably empathic approach to how they practice medicine.

Portrait of a Suicidal Physician

There is no unitary presentation of a physician who might be acutely suicidal, but the description in Table 11–4 (in the absence of DSM-IV-TR nosology), which is a composite of scores of suicidal physicians we have treated, captures some of the cardinal symptoms.

TABLE 11–4.   A suicidal physician

- Highly anxious, worried, despondent, sad, flat, or numb—this may be reported as both a subjective state and an observable picture by the family, colleagues, and treating physician.

- Not sleeping, especially with middle and terminal insomnia—the physician awakens with a low mood and dread of facing the day.

- Weakness, tiredness, and an inner sense of feeling much older than one's years.

- Anorexia and weight loss, or weight loss without a true loss of appetite— the physician reports that he or she is "worrying" the weight off.

- Cognitive slowing, word-finding difficulty, inability to concentrate, forgetfulness, and poor recent memory—the physician worries about a dementing illness.

- Panic attacks that are a separate phenomena or layered on generalized anxiety—the physician feels as though he or she is going crazy and will be hallucinating soon.

- Obsessive ruminations—some physicians use this language or describe themselves as "churning."

- Somatic symptoms—many physicians are worried or are convinced (suggesting delusional depression) that they have some undiagnosed, rare, or mysterious medical illness that explains their bodily symptoms.

- Despairing and hopeless thinking—they often fear that they will not respond to treatment, that they will not survive this illness, or that they will never practice medicine again.

- Thoughts of suicide (passive and active) with a wish for death—they may be both planning suicide and rehearsing the plan. Suicidal thinking may be frightening at first but with progression to a plan for enactment, patients become calmer. Given the need that physicians have for autonomy, some severely depressed physicians are comforted by their plans for ending their lives.

When a Physician Is at Imminent Risk for Suicide

Simon (2006) argued that *imminence* is a euphemism for short-term prediction and that the term imposes an illusory time frame on an unpredictable act. It is better to think of risk factors for suicide that require careful assessment. With that spirit in mind, physicians may be at high risk for self-harm when one or more of the following are present:

- *Severe agitation and unrestrained restlessness.* These states may be due to the illness worsening or due to side effects of medication, whether prescribed by a physician or self-prescribed.
- *Impulsivity.* This may be de novo in a physician who has rarely been impulsive or may be longstanding and associated with the physician's personality, alcohol or street drug use, or attention-deficit/hyperactive disorder.
- *Mixed mood states in rapidly cycling bipolar illness.* This may be a psychiatric emergency and require expert psychopharmacological consultation and care (including protection) to prevent the physician from harming him- or herself.
- *Emerging early psychosis with ideas of reference and paranoid thinking.* This is terrifying and may precipitate frenetic action on the part of the physician.
- *Disinhibiting effects of alcohol and other drugs.* It is well documented that the vast majority of suicide attempters and victims of suicide have ingested chemicals (Mack and Lightdale 2006).
- *Very recent "last straw" trigger.* Examples include a relationship breakup, loss of custody of children or of visiting privileges, a charge of professional misconduct with a patient resulting in extreme humiliation and fear of public scrutiny.
- *A sudden and proximal calm and peaceful state of mind.* In other words, the physician has a carefully considered suicide plan and is now at peace because he or she knows the end of suffering is near.

Assessment and Treatment of the Suicidal Physician

One of the cardinal rules for psychiatrists who are assessing and treating physicians is never to compromise one's clinical judgment simply because the patient is a physician. There is a long and wrenching history of physician-patients killing themselves because they were underdiagnosed, undertreated, and not hospitalized voluntarily or involuntarily for safety. The treating psychiatrist, albeit well intentioned, succumbed to the patient's concerns about privacy and image (or projected his or her own conflicts about these matters onto the patient) and did not adequately protect the patient from self-harm. With this background, here are some basic principles to consider when assessing and treating physicians who are, or may be, suicidal.

1. *Try to assess physicians as quickly as possible, especially self-referrals from physicians themselves.* When physicians telephone psychiatrists directly, they may downplay how sick they are or may legitimately not know the degree of illness. It is well known that physicians delay seeking help for myriad reasons that we have discussed earlier in this book. They may need to be seen later

the same day, necessitating a form of professional courtesy—that is, the psychiatrist stays late to accommodate a colleague. Attempting to gauge the degree of urgency over the telephone, some psychiatrists ask the caller if he or she is suicidal. Even if they are, many physicians find the question jarring and thus will not be honest and disclose something so personal—and serious—over the phone (Myers 1996b). It is prudent to see the caller quickly and to err on the side of safety and caution.

2. *Take any reference that a physician-patient makes to suicide very seriously.* Physicians may be oblique and raise the matter in philosophical, abstract, and intellectual terms as though to engage the treating physician in a dialogue or debate. Some physicians may mention the suicide or suicide attempt of one of their patients, but they are actually hinting at their own suicidality. Always inquire about methods and means of suicide. Given that overdose is a common means in physicians, ask about stashed pills at home, whether prescribed or otherwise. Ask physicians in critical care medicine, emergency medicine, anesthesia, and surgery about such drugs as potassium chloride, insulin, barbiturates, lidocaine, digoxin, and fentanyl. Ask psychiatrists about hording tricyclic antidepressants, lithium, or monoamine oxidase inhibitors. Ask all physicians about firearms.

3. *Listen carefully with attention and sensitivity—and vigilance—to physicians who are very ill and have many of the symptoms described earlier but who deny that they are suicidal.* As with deeply depressed lay patients who tell their psychiatrist "I could never kill myself; I can't do that to my wife and kids," note their denial but return to this statement again because the patient can worsen and begin to feel burdensome. He or she may come to view death as a relief to his or her family.

4. *Assume, for all intents and purposes, that all physicians have contemplated suicide—along a huge continuum from minimally or rarely to seriously and often.* This is partly because they are physicians and have treated suicidal patients at some point in their training and career, irrespective of their branch of medicine. In addition, most physicians know how to kill themselves. In fact, physicians who feel free to be candid with their psychiatrist not uncommonly state "I know how to kill myself; don't all doctors? And I know how to do it right. I don't want to do a half-assed job and be disabled; I've looked after too many botched attempts in my work as a doctor." These are strong words, but the treating psychiatrist need not panic if his or her patient is not acutely suicidal. What the patient is describing is taking control over one's life and death if the treatment does not work.

5. *Appreciate why physician-patients who are suicidal may not be completely candid with their psychiatrist.* They are very aware that the psychiatrist has the ability and power to overrule their reticence about or refusal to come into the hospital voluntarily. They know that inpatient hospitalization means having to take medication, or higher dosages of medication, including antipsychot-

ics, orally or by injection. They may require electroconvulsive therapy. They have to abide by a prescribed daily program. They have to surrender their medical license temporarily. They worry about their privacy. These kinds of rules and losses are very tough for physicians who are used to independence and freedom and who prefer to give orders rather than follow those of others. However, they may be pleasantly surprised at the help they receive, as in this first-person account:

> I was spiraling downward so fast that I couldn't slow the agitation down and counter the growing isolation from others. For me, psychiatric hospitalization was a godsend. It took a monumental weight off my shoulders....the weight of the fear of acting on suicidal thoughts. I was not treated as a VIP. I formed sincere and caring relationships with other inpatients, a special sort of bond that is not usually seen by the ward psychiatrist or staff. The other patients knew I was a physician and a psychiatrist, and I made an effort to just be a patient, not a psychiatrist. They treated me with respect and concern.[1]

6. *When a psychiatric inpatient stay is necessary, try to hospitalize physician-patients in a setting where they are not on staff or otherwise affiliated with the institution.* This may be easier said than done, especially in small communities. The arguments for this recommendation are that physician-patients will not have to worry about their privacy and confidentiality and that the treating staff will not be in any conflict-of-interest situation. Boundaries will be clear: the person is a patient, not someone with whom there is a preexisting relationship. The arguments against are that sometimes physician-patients in academic settings have access to psychiatric experts who may be the best ones to look after them. If they fear that a more distant setting is inferior, this should be taken into account. Similarly, if the patient is already in treatment and has an established relationship with a psychiatrist whom he or she respects, the transfer may not work. Well-intentioned decisions by the treating psychiatrist may be misunderstood by deeply depressed and regressed physician-patients. The patient feels abandoned and burdensome, and his or her already lowered self-worth is reduced further. Feelings of isolation may also be increased if the distance is prohibitive and family and friends can visit rarely, if at all (Bauman 1995).

7. *When hospitalizing suicidal residents, make every effort to reassure them about their having a treatable illness and being able to return to training when well.* They are usually very nervous about breaches of confidentiality to their fel-

---

[1]Mark Dembert, M.D., M.P.H.: "A Psychiatrist Speaks About Being Hospitalized in the Early 1990s," unpublished personal communication, August 26, 2007. Reprinted with permission.

low residents and beyond. They do not know the limitations of confidentiality beyond their training director and dean of postgraduate education. They worry that they will be marked for life and that career doors will close. Unlike physicians who are older or at a different career stage, they do not have the experience in medicine to have had colleagues in similar circumstances who recovered from their illnesses and are now back working and enjoying life. The number of residents whose illness is so refractory to treatment that they must abandon their professional goals is quite small.

8. *Treat sleep difficulties aggressively with appropriate medication.* Many suicidal physicians newly admitted to hospital have not been sleeping well on the outside, and because of the strong association between poor sleep and suicidal behavior, this should be treated aggressively with appropriate medication. Similarly, because unrelenting anxiety and agitation can lead to impulsivity, these states require immediate psychopharmacological attention as well.

9. *With any physician-patient who is reluctant to give permission for collateral information gathering, be persistent in a supportive and exacting way.* They can be reassured about privacy and confidentiality. One must emphasize that this information is needed to have a completely comprehensive assessment. One strategy that can be effective is to appeal to the physician's own sense of basic values, in the name of good medical practice, that collaborative information from family members and/or previous treating professionals is essential.

Treating the Suicidal Physician on an Ambulatory Basis

Not all physician-patients who report suicidal thinking will require hospitalization. In fact, unless they are in an acute crisis, physicians with borderline personality who have supports in place and an ongoing therapeutic relationship may be worsened by hospitalization. That diagnosis aside, there are also physicians in various stages of recovery from a mood disorder who can be managed safely outside of hospital. The context is physician-like vigilance. One or more family members can accompany the patient to the psychiatrists's office and provide updates of improved or worsening symptoms or function. The treating psychiatrist should not hesitate to revise the treatment and admit to hospital any suicidal physician whose risk of self-harm has increased. A written or oral suicide prevention contract, or "no-harm contract," should never be substituted for a careful clinical assessment (American Psychiatric Association 2004).

Psychodynamic treatment can be employed with suicidal patients, including physicians. Because this work is difficult for psychiatrists, it is best embarked upon in a series of deliberate, carefully placed steps (Gabbard and Allison 2006; see Table 11–5).

TABLE 11–5. Steps in the psychodynamic treatment of the suicidal patient

---

- Establish a therapeutic alliance.

- Differentiate between the fantasy and the act of suicide.

- Discuss the limits of treatment.

- Investigate precipitating events.

- Explore fantasies of the interpersonal impact of suicide.

- Establish level of suicidality present at baseline.

- Monitor transference and countertransference.

Source. Reprinted from Gabbard GO, Allison SE: "Psychodynamic Treatment," in *The American Psychiatric Publishing Textbook of Suicide Assessment and Management.* Edited by Simon RI, Hales RE. Washington, DC, American Psychiatric Publishing, 2006. Used with permission.

Gabbard and Allison (2006) highlight the centrality of a good therapeutic alliance, and achieving this should be possible with most physician-patients. They also emphasize the task of distinguishing between the patient's fantasy of suicide and a true intention to act. For some the fantasy of escape keeps them going. The therapist must be explicit that he or she cannot prevent the physician from committing suicide, and there must be a clear differentiation between the therapist's and the patient's responsibilities within the confines of the therapeutic alliance. Any stressful triggers to suicidal behavior must be explored, as well as the patient's sense of the impact of his or her death by suicide. Additional steps include (with chronically suicidal patients) recording a baseline index of suicidality so that any worsening can be detected. At all times, the therapist must monitor transference and countertransference.

A few words about countertransference are important in this context. Most therapists worry a good deal when treating suicidal patients, especially if those patients are physicians. This anxiety may range from mild to overwhelming. Overinvestment in preventing suicide at all costs may shut the patient down, precipitate acting out, and even spark a suicide attempt or death by suicide. Well-intentioned statements about medication changes, hospitalization, and involuntary admission to hospital may be perceived by the physician-patient as threats. The therapist may feel anger and rage at the patient for giving up, for not getting better, or for wanting to die. Therapists may struggle with accepting feelings of failure, guilt, or shame when patients attempt suicide or die by suicide. Some feel that their help has been rejected and that they have been rendered impotent. They may imagine that colleagues think they have "screwed up." Finally, intellectualization is a common defense used by therapists to ward off many of the conflicted feelings associated with treatment of suicidal physicians. Supervision can be very helpful for therapists engaged in this kind of treatment, and we highly recommend it.

Maltsberger (2006) outlined some fundamental steps in the outpatient treatment of suicidal patients. Some of these are 1) complete a thorough suicide risk assessment at the beginning and keep it up-to-date; 2) obtain informed consent and a risk-benefit analysis; 3) only accept patients who are willing to commit to staying alive and give treatment a chance; 4) ensure that inpatient admission is possible on short notice; 5) note what the patient's support resources are; 6) make certain that the patient does not control the treatment; and 7) keep good records. In an earlier article Maltsberger (2001) called for an emotionally full and active engagement of the therapist with the patient. He underscored the real relationship, not the transference, and emphasized that the therapist must be available to the patient as a sturdy, reliable object with whom to identify. Furthermore, the therapist's attitude must be caring, not neutral. The therapeutic alliance is built upon the therapist's commitment to the patient's growth and the regaining of self-sustaining attributes. Maltsberger's recommendations are particularly relevant to the treatment of suicidal physicians. They not only expect this kind of approach from another health professional but also can identify because they themselves are physicians.

Any previously suicidal physician who is now well and who is ready to go back to work should be returning on a graduated basis only and should be monitored closely over the first few weeks. Many physicians (for various reasons) pressure their psychiatrists to consent to their resuming work, sometimes sooner than they should. Mood certainty, stability, and sleep can be lost quickly if the physician works too many hours in a stressful setting after being on medical leave. Anxiety, loss of confidence, disappointment in one's self, and a resurgence of self-destructive thinking ensue.

Aftermath of Physician Suicide

Despite best efforts at suicide assessment and treatment, suicides can and do occur in clinical practice. It is estimated that 50% of psychiatrists will lose at least one patient to suicide over the course of their career, and this loss is deemed among the most difficult professional experiences encountered by a psychiatrist (American Psychiatric Association 2004). In one study (Chemtob et al. 1988), approximately half of the psychiatrists who had lost a patient to suicide experienced stress levels comparable with those of people recovering from the death of a parent. There is now a significant literature on the impact of suicide on mental health professionals (Campbell 2006; Gitlin 1999, 2006; Hendin et al. 2000; Myers and Fine 2006) but very little published on the loss of a physician-patient to suicide (Myers 1995, 1998; Shneidman 2004).

Because of identification or perceived judgment by the patient's medical colleagues, psychiatrists who lose a physician-patient to suicide may feel even more stressed. If it is widely known in the medical community (or beyond) that the physician died by suicide as well as the identity of the treater, the psychiatrist may feel exposed, judged, and perhaps violated. These feelings may compound the host of emotions and thoughts (shock, grief, guilt, shame, anger, symptoms of posttraumatic stress disorder, and diminished professional self-confidence) that the psychiatrist is already experiencing. Individuals should not hesitate to seek support for themselves. Safeguarding patient confidentiality always and protecting details, the psychiatrist can benefit from the support of family, friends, medical colleagues, clergypersons, and so forth. Seeking psychotherapy can also be very helpful at this time. Notifying one's liability insurance carrier regarding risk management appraisal of the case and contacting an attorney (if there are concerns about litigation) are also helpful self-care strategies.

Some mental health professionals are uncertain or ambivalent about attending the funeral, visitation, or memorial service of their deceased patient. Although the decision is basically an individual preferential one, there are arguments for and against. Some individuals attend for personal reasons (it is helpful for their own mourning) and professional reasons (there is an honoring of and respect for the patient and his or her family). Being present also provides a chance to offer professional support to the family in the ensuing days or weeks. They may offer to assist the family themselves or to facilitate referrals to colleagues or other community resources. The major argument against attending a service is the situation in which the treating professional is not welcome—that is, the survivors have very negative feelings (including anger and blame) toward the individual, and his or her presence would be deemed inappropriate or intrusive. It is best to check first before appearing.

Whether he or she attends a service of remembrance or not, the treating health professional should not hesitate to contact the survivors (Campbell 2006). It is well known that survivors of suicide are more vulnerable to physical and psychological disorders (Myers and Fine 2006) and are at an increased risk of suicide themselves. Conversations with family members can be appropriate and can allay grief and assist them in obtaining help (American Psychiatric Association 2004). This is largely for humanitarian reasons, but there is a risk management benefit as well. Expressions of condolence, sadness, sympathy, or regret for the patient's death are known to play some role in reducing the risk of being sued. Attorneys advise, however, that under no circumstances should the treating professional disclose any confidential material of the patient's treatment nor make self-incriminating or self-exonerating statements to the family.

Interviews with survivors, including the families of physicians who died by suicide, are almost universally well received (Fine 1997). Even a single visit with the treating professional (or team if the loved one was hospitalized) provides

---

TABLE 11–6.   Reactions of the deceased physician's colleagues

- Mourning—full range of emotions and thoughts

- Systemic anxiety—personal vulnerability, contagion fears, who's next?

- Guilt and blame—at self and others for not doing more, missing clues, not reaching out, failing the physician colleague

- Anger and rage at the deceased—for "giving up," being "selfish," leaving his or her family, abandoning his or her patients, "dumping" more work on those left behind, tainting the public perception of physicians as invincible

- Business as usual—calm, cool demeanor, defensive intellectualization and rationalization, "suicide is just an occupational hazard when you're a doctor"

---

some relief to the innumerable (and often unanswerable) questions as well as some clarity, ballast, and hope. Measured self-disclosures by the therapist help: "Your brother was a good man—he fought a tough battle"; "Your daughter lived with dignity"; "Like you, I too have wondered if your husband's loss of his medical license when he relapsed and started using cocaine was completely overwhelming for him"; "She was a wonderful physician, so loved by her patients and colleagues. I will miss her too."

When a physician dies by suicide and his or her family members are non-medical or unsophisticated about psychiatric illness, the treating psychiatrist can be helpful in a very unique way. There is a perception that physicians have it all: a profession, challenging work, prestige, intelligence, success, and most of all money and its trappings (Myers 2006). Having so much, why would a doctor take his or her own life? Central to the incredulity is that a major tenet of the calling to medicine is to preserve and protect life. Isn't that why men and women become doctors? When physicians kill themselves, it is very frightening and disorienting. "If they've given up on life, what's it say for the rest of us?" is the refrain. By providing some elementary psychoeducation about depression or other relevant illness, the treating psychiatrist can offer the family much solace.

Finally, there is another way that psychiatrists can help in the aftermath of physician suicide. When a doctor in the psychiatrist's hometown or nearby community dies by suicide, and that physician was not a patient of the psychiatrist, he or she can offer to meet with the grieving physician (or more expansively, health professional) community. Historically, physician suicides were covered up, denied, whispered about, and not addressed openly and collectively by colleagues. Today, with more knowledge and less stigma, medical communities are facing and confronting these tragic deaths of their colleagues. Within days of the death, a psychiatrist, especially at arm's length, can act as a facilitator when these professionals come together in a forum to talk. Tables 11–6 and 11–7 outline what to expect and how one can help.

TABLE 11–7.   Roles and responsibilities of the facilitator

- Welcome everyone for coming and being together at such a difficult time; acknowledge the profound emotions that suicide triggers.

- Make a statement urging all present to respect and protect everyone's confidentiality and privacy about anything said in the meeting.

- Invite any or all to speak as they feel comfortable.

- Encourage ventilation and airing of myriad feelings and thoughts.

- Try not to judge; remember that all health professionals are human beings first, and they are in the acute stages of grief and their emotions are very raw, even primitive.

- Succinctly address questions posed about parameters of grief, what to say to the grieving family, what to expect after suicide, treatment resources, and more, but revert back to the group so others can open up—avoid a mini-lecture.

- Encourage discussion about any creative ideas the group has about ways of remembering their colleague—a plaque, memorial lecture, trust fund, donation, striking a small committee to explore options.

- Volunteer to give a grand rounds after a few months, if they wish, on physician health and self-care.

Key Points

- Studies on physicians' suicide collectively show modestly elevated rates for men and highly elevated rates for women.

- Postulated reasons for elevated rates of suicide in physicians include susceptibility to mood and substance use disorders, perfectionistic and self-critical personality traits, stigma, knowledge of toxicology, and ready access to drugs.

- Psychiatrists must never let their clinical judgment be influenced by the fact that their patient is a physician. Suicidal physicians deserve state-of-the-art care and must be treated like any suicidal individual.

- Stigma in the house of medicine is pervasive and toxic and must be addressed and confronted so that physicians living with unrecognized, untreated, self-treated, or undertreated psychiatric illnesses can come forward for lifesaving care.

- Psychiatrists who lose a physician-patient to suicide may be severely stressed and should avail themselves of all possible supports. This enables the psychiatrist to be more helpful and effective with the families of their deceased patient.

- Psychiatrists can assist medical communities that are mourning the loss of a physician colleague to suicide by facilitating groups of health professionals who have come together.

Prevention

The task of conceptualizing a "prevention plan" is overwhelming, to say the least. To begin with, we must ask, "prevention of what?" The types of problems recounted in this book are diverse and cannot be reduced to a simple formula that can be applied in "cookie cutter" fashion. The perfectionism that leads to burnout, for example, is a different problem than the identification of corrupt medical students. Detecting antisocial individuals may help us weed out predator types who may commit sexual boundary violations with patients, but it will not be very useful in protecting hyperresponsible physicians from themselves. Similarly, a program designed to prevent suicide is not the same as one that implements prophylactic measures for marital conflict. Some physicians are particularly susceptible to alcoholism, whereas others may have short tempers and blow up at colleagues in the workplace. Each of the psychiatric disorders that are considered in this book have complex etiologies involving genetic vulnerability and environmental factors. Thus knowing at what point and how to intervene requires both a breadth of knowledge of complex conditions and a creative approach to preventive medicine—a rare combination. To further complicate matters, many medical students, residents, and young physicians are convinced that none of the difficulties described in this volume will ever happen to them, and they may go through the motions of preventive efforts without ever internalizing the seriousness of their own risk. Finally, the culture of medicine may question the value of taking time out for reflection and self-care. Such time is time spent away from one's work.

Nevertheless, a number of measures can be spelled out for consideration when thinking about the large morbidity related to physician psychology and the stresses of medical practice. We start by looking at the admissions procedure to medical school, then training itself, and then the postresidency period wherein physicians navigate the vicissitudes of medical practice and encounter the stresses faced by mature professionals.

Selection of Medical Students

A long-standing problem in the screening of medical school applicants is that cognitive capacities are overvalued. Cumulative grade point average and the Medical College Admissions Test (MCAT) provide concrete, quantitative data to measure the cognitive capabilities of a potential student. These capacities are measured in numbers and therefore are much easier to assess than the noncognitive skills, such as empathy, compassion, creativity, the capacity to solve difficult clinical problems, and interpersonal sensitivity. Moreover, admissions committees know that the *U.S. News & World Report* rankings include the grade point average and MCAT scores of entering students. It seems not to matter that such rankings are derived from a nonscientific survey of deans, department chairs, and assorted professors. Medical school deans live and die by such rankings, however arbitrary, and often place pressure on admissions committees to select the best and the brightest based purely on these cognitive measures (Wagoner 2006). Hence the stereotype of the premedical student who is a driven, compulsive high-achiever with little life experience is exactly the type of applicant who is likely to succeed.

These qualities do not necessarily predict whether an applicant may be capable of thinking—that is, creative enough to come up with novel solutions to complex problems in a clinical setting. In addition, one can be outstanding on objective tests but completely lacking in empathy. In fact, empathy scores are closely linked to ratings of clinical competence but have been found to have no linkage to the performance on objective examinations such as the MCAT, first- and second-year grade point averages, or even scores on the Step 1 of the United States Medical Licensing Examination (Hojat et al. 2002). The student's genuine interest in medicine and motivation to care for others in a compassionate way are also not measured by cognitive scores (Wagoner 2006).

The noncognitive measures used for admission to medical schools in the United States include interviews, personal statements, letters of recommendation, and supplemental application forms. The letters of recommendation are uniformly positive and "by the numbers" to a large extent, so they rarely say much of use for the admissions committee. Interviews may be revealing, but research has failed to demonstrate that interview data are reliable or valid (Albanese et al. 2003).

Antisocial applicants who have a corrupt character are notorious for being able to convince interviewers that they are entirely normal (Gabbard 2005a). Personal statements are often crafted with the help of others who know what an admissions committee is looking for and thus may similarly be limited in their value. Screening out corrupt or antisocial individuals may require a search for a criminal record or phone conversations with key people in the applicant's undergraduate college. This process is labor intensive and may turn up minimal data, so it is often bypassed.

Wagoner (2006) suggested a number of changes that may help the medical school admission screening process to achieve greater balance, more breadth in terms of diversity, and a greater number of creative students. These suggestions include the following:

- Reach agreement among medical schools to assign greater weight to noncognitive strengths.
- Establish a freer range of MCAT scores and grade point averages for new students.
- Modify personal statements to specifically identify areas that must be addressed by each student.
- Make the personal statement sufficiently complex that companies or entrepreneurial individuals cannot simply devise answers for students and sell them to potential applicants.
- Develop trained interviewers in a standardized format.
- Fund further research on how criteria for admissions predict success in medical school.

One salient fact that must be squarely addressed, however, is that it is impossible to prevent all the problems of physicians, even with the most sophisticated screening process imaginable. The gatekeeping function of medical school admissions committees is only one small factor among a host that must be considered.

Emphasizing Professionalism in Medical School

As we noted in Chapter 3 ("Psychiatric Evaluation of Physicians"), professionalism was once absent from medical schools and residency training. Much has changed in the past few decades; professionalism is now considered one of the core competencies in medical education. The fundamental principles of ethical medical practice—devotion to the patient instead of oneself, sensitive treatment of colleagues and coworkers, and observation of professional boundaries in the workplace—need to be inculcated in medical school, both through didactic teaching and through the internalization of role models who teach medical students in clinical settings.

The wisdom of training all students in professionalism has gained a good deal of support from a landmark study published in the *New England Journal of Medicine* on the disciplinary action dispensed by medical boards and its linkage to medical school behavior (Papadakis et al. 2005). In this investigation, 740 violations among 235 physicians leading to disciplinary action from 40 state medical boards were studied. Unprofessional behavior was the leading cause of disciplinary action in these cases, and the following subtypes were catalogued:

- Alcohol or drug abuse
- Unprofessional conduct
- Criminal conviction
- Negligence
- Prescribing of controlled substances in an inappropriate manner
- Sexual misconduct
- Failure to conform to minimal standards of acceptable medical practice
- Violation of a board law or order or of probation
- Failure to meet requirements for continuing medical education
- Fraudulent or inappropriate billing practices
- Failure to maintain adequate medical records
- Failure to report adverse actions against one's self in accordance with board rules
- Conduct that might defraud or harm the public

The 235 graduates came from three medical schools that were geographically distributed, and their discipline from the 40 state medical boards occurred between 1990 and 2003. This cohort was matched with 460 control physicians chosen according to medical school and graduation year. Medical school records were examined to yield predictor variables, including narratives describing unprofessional behavior, standardized test scores, grades, and demographic characteristics.

When the results were analyzed, disciplinary action by a medical board was strongly associated with unprofessional behavior during medical school. Those forms of unprofessional behavior most strongly linked with disciplinary action were severe irresponsibility and severely diminished capacity for self-improvement. Although there was some connection between disciplinary action and low scores on the MCAT and poor grades in the basic science years of medical schools, these linkages were much weaker than those of unprofessional behavior. Male gender was not found to be a risk factor.

As a result of these findings, the authors of the study suggested that standardized instruments should be implemented to assess personal qualities of medical school applicants. They also strongly advocate for improved systems of evaluation in medical school that carefully monitor professional behavior. Too often such evaluation is done in a perfunctory manner. Students need feedback to know what areas require improvement.

When professionalism items are identified in medical school, remediation is essential if we are to prevent future disciplinary actions. One of the lessons of the Papadakis study is that much of this behavior is ingrained in character and will be longstanding and repetitive throughout one's career. Too often, instances of unprofessional behavior are ignored or dismissed as "difficulties in learning." When misconduct is taken seriously and disciplinary action is threatened, certain medical students will hire an attorney to intimidate progression committees or deans. The threat of litigation may cause some medical school officials to back down and find a way to graduate the student rather than to face a lengthy and costly lawsuit. An independent psychiatric evaluation, such as those described in Chapter 3, may be essential to diagnose psychopathology and to design an optimal remediation or treatment plan tailored to the student. An assessment may also determine whether the student should be dismissed from the medical school because of severe personality pathology rather than be allowed to progress to graduation.

Didactic seminars that teach ethics, professional boundaries, and the basic principles of professionalism are useful and essential in medical school education. However, medical students often express the feeling that they "already know this stuff" and allow their minds to wander in class or skip class altogether. Hence the main thrust of professionalism education occurs in the clinics and hospital wards where influential teachers demonstrate how they relate to patients with respect and sensitivity.

> Dr. Mannheim was a professor of obstetrics and gynecology in a Midwestern medical school who trained medical students in an adolescent outpatient clinic at a major teaching hospital. On the first day of the rotation, Professor Mannheim explained to the medical students, "These adolescents are deserving of our respect and consideration, even though they are socially and economically deprived and in the middle of a life crisis involving a teenage pregnancy. I do not want to hear 'Get your butt down, honey' or any other demeaning phrases echoing through this clinic. Treat them as you would want your own family members to be treated by colleagues." Dr. Mannheim then demonstrated the professionalism he was advocating by seeing some of the patients himself, with four medical students in tow. All of the patients were addressed as "Ms. Smith" or "Ms. Jones" and given ample time to ask questions and explain their concerns to Professor Mannheim. Pelvic examination was explained in detail to them, and they were given the opportunity to ask for clarifications if the procedure was not clearly understood.

The kind of role-modeling reflected in Dr. Mannheim's clinic is not easy to achieve in a busy academic center where clinicians are increasingly expected to generate revenues for the department in which they work. Many faculty members rush through rounds and examinations to try to increase revenues. Many of them were trained in an era in which professionalism was neglected, and they may actually model behavior that is damaging to professionalism.

> Dr. Bradley taught physical diagnosis to two second-year medical students during his rounds in a teaching hospital. He was known to be a brilliant cardiologist, but his manner of relating to female coworkers was a source of considerable concern among hospital employees. On rounds with his two students one morning, he entered a patient room and found a student nurse helping the patient eat breakfast. She asked Dr. Bradley if he wanted the patient on her back. Dr. Bradley retorted, "No, I want you on your back" and laughed heartily. Neither medical student found it funny, and neither laughed. They later discussed whether they should file a complaint against Dr. Bradley. After considerable discussion, they decided against it because they feared retribution from Dr. Bradley.

Although this vignette is extreme in its lack of professionalism, it is not uncommon for role models to engage in egregious behavior. Many feel they have earned the right to behave however they like and that others should tolerate it. These behaviors can ultimately be transmitted from one generation to another.

The informal experiences that medical students have in their clinical assignments are often referred to as the "hidden curriculum" in professionalism education (Stern and Papadakis 2006). To a large extent, this hidden curriculum involving routines, rules, and regulations is transmitted as much by residents as by faculty, often late at night when students are on call with the resident on their service. Medical students in that situation observe residents behaving in ways that create a lasting impression: How a family member is told that a relative has died; how a resident talks to a patient about a procedure that needs to be done; or how a physical examination is conducted in a respectful manner.

Part of teaching professionalism is to encourage the expansion of the capacity to mentalize. Again and again, physicians come to evaluation because they have not made the effort to empathize with how others feel in their interactions with them. This obliviousness or lack of mentalization may extend to family members, patients, colleagues, and allied health professionals working with them in a hospital or clinic. Physicians are frequently unaware that when they don the white coat, they are suddenly in a position of power. Moreover, patients experience them as a transference figure that has parental qualities. Hence they overvalue what the physician says and may be terrified of disagreeing or not going along with what the physician recommends. Good mentalizing overlaps with sensitive empathy to others, so it is a skill that is central to the doctor–patient relationship.

The hidden curriculum must be supplemented by the formal teaching of medical educators. Clarity about professional expectations is essential. The rationale for them should be explained as well as the consequences of not living up to these expectations.

Although we have focused on the types of individuals who become medical students, the role modeling necessary while in training, and teaching professionalism to prevent behavior problems down the road, there are other preventive measures that address health and well-being of students. Many medical schools offer one to several days of orientation for entering medical students. The prototype of this is the Health Awareness Workshop (Dickstein 1998) introduced at the University of Louisville in 1981 but now incorporated in many medical schools throughout North America. Over a span of 4 days, incoming medical students participate in workshops and seminars (co-led by faculty and senior students) that address diet, exercise, stress, studying, recreation, self-care, peer support, recognition of psychological distress and psychiatric illness, spirituality, marriage, and family. Other schools offer experiential workshops on dealing with harassment and abuse, the use of SOS (Students Offering Support), awareness of alcohol and other drug use and abuse, improving study habits and efficiency, outreach to gay and lesbian students, and accessing medical and counseling services on and off campus (Myers 2000).

Promoting Balance in Residency Training

In our consideration of prevention, the separation of medical school and residency is arbitrary in the sense that the culture of medicine instills similar values in both medical students and residents. More responsibility is given to residents, of course, and this change in and of itself places more stress on the developing physician. Much of the stress of residency is attributed to long hours of work. However, as we noted in Chapter 1 ("The Psychology of Physicians and the Culture of Medicine"), that explanation is oversimplified. In the 2006 study of 4,015 interns in U.S. residency programs, Landrigan et al. (2006) found that after mandatory limits to work hours were imposed, 83% of the interns were noncompliant for at least 1 month in the year following their introduction. In other words, one can attempt to change work hours, but the culture of medicine and the characterological disposition of residents leads them to work extended shifts anyway. Moreover, Gelfand et al. (2004) conducted a longitudinal study comparing surgery residents' self-reported work hours and burnout scores 1 week before and 6 months after the 2003 Accreditation Council for Graduate Medical Education 80-hour work week restriction was implemented. Although the work hours decreased significantly, mean burnout scores did not. In fact, depersonalization, often a sign of burnout, increased from 56% to 70%.

Neither sleep deprivation nor work hours alone are associated with reduction in burnout of residents (Thomas 2004). Instead, the intensity of the work experience during the day for the resident and the extent to which that work interferes with the resident's home life appear to be more strongly linked to resident burnout. Restoring balance between work and home lives thus may be critically important in preventing burnout, depression, and demoralization. Because work habits are established in residency training, future burnout may be headed off as well. Other factors that may improve resident well-being may be facilitating supportive interactions among peers, increasing one's control of work hours, and helping residents prioritize.

Peer support may be critically important in the training setting when one makes an error. In Chapter 1 we described the vicious circle of personal distress and decreased empathy associated with self-perceived errors. These factors lead to further perceived errors in the future. It is reasonable to assume that this cycle can be influenced by turning to peers for support rather than retreating into isolation (O'Reilly 2006). The culture of medicine may regard a physician who turns to others for support after an error as weak or dependent—not in keeping with the "Lone Ranger" mentality of the medical culture. According to this ethos, one should shrug off adverse experiences and keep moving. Some hospitals and healthcare systems have instituted a structured peer support team to assist colleagues when something goes wrong in clinical work (O'Reilly 2006). Similarly, some psychiatric departments have instituted faculty teams to intervene with residents after a patient's suicide.

Abuse of residents has been identified as a significant stressor during training, and its diminution or eradication is critical (Myers 1996a). The effects of abuse are well documented and include anger, fear, depression, irritability, feelings of humiliation and alienation, a sense of helplessness, and many physical symptoms. Some victimized residents meet criteria for posttraumatic stress disorder. Educating residents about this subject, teaching recognition and coping strategies, and identifying perpetrators quickly and dealing with them smartly are all examples of preventive measures that work.

Self-Monitoring

In discussing preventive measures that promote physician health, we must realistically face the fact that the culture of medicine will change only incrementally, and much of the impetus for prevention must come from within the self. Hence self-monitoring by physicians is imperative in heading off burnout, depression, family strife, drug and alcohol abuse, and suicidal despair.

The freshly minted physician who leaves residency or fellowship and goes into private practice, an academic position, or other institutional work will experience an absence of external validation in a way that can be highly disconcerting. After having been in training for many years, one is used to receiving feedback on one's performance, both informally through comments from supervisors and formally through performance evaluations. It can be jarring when one has "grown up" professionally and is no longer rewarded with the approval of older colleagues in a parental role. This absence may be especially felt if one is in a private practice setting that is relatively isolated. In perfectionistic physicians, this thundering silence can activate the concern that one is not working hard enough.

When physicians seek validation from their patients, they encounter another set of difficulties. Certain patients are characterologically predisposed to be dissatisfied with treatment, no matter how good it is. The physician is a transference figure who may become the target of the bitterness and resentment associated with a parent who was never sufficiently attentive. The caring physician will raise hopes in some patients that will ultimately be dashed. Physicians are often bearers of bad news. Thus although some patients will offer validation, others will accuse the physician of a host of sins. Depending exclusively on patients to maintain one's self-esteem is a recipe for trouble.

The childhood conviction that perfection is the root to receiving validation, approval, and love may take hold and cause a physician to work longer hours and more compulsively to prove that he or she is worthy of being a physician responsible for the lives of others. Physicians at whatever level of experience must accept the fact that they cannot please everyone. They will always have angry and disgruntled patients. There will always be colleagues who are competitive and try to work harder than anyone. These physicians will always be disappointed in others who lack the same work ethic. Spouses and children will also feel upset with their physician spouse or parent from time to time because life and death matters may call the physician away. It is simply impossible to balance work and family perfectly.

Hence physicians who attempt to practice self-care and the balancing of work and family will inevitably make others unhappy to some extent. Nevertheless, all physicians might usefully participate in an exercise to monitor the way one uses one's time (Gabbard and Menninger 1988).

> On a sheet of paper, rank order your priorities in life. Be as honest as possible in listing what you regard as the five most important activities in your life. Then take out your schedule book from last week and examine whether the way you spent your time reflects the priorities you value in your life.

Most physicians will find that they have allowed themselves to be sucked into a vortex of work demands that have insidiously taken over their lives so they feel they have very little control over how they spend their time. Reordering their priorities may require change that irritates others or may even require moving to a different work setting. The critical point in this exercise, however, is this:

Every physician is making an active choice about how time is spent. Not making a choice is also a choice.

Physicians frequently lack a sense of agency; they feel "put upon" by others and feel powerless to do anything about it. The demands of patients, their colleagues, the institution, the department chair, or external agencies appear to drive their lives in a direction that leads to chronic discontent.

Monitoring of the self also entails observing how one copes with the stress of medical practice. How important does a drink before dinner become? How much wine does one drink with dinner? Does one drink more on weekends? Is self-medication through samples the way one copes with a bad day? Does one feel ashamed about one's behavior after attending a party?

Some physicians simply work harder when they begin to feel beleaguered. Self-monitoring may help one realize that problems cannot be solved in isolation. Physicians need to make a practice of reaching out to peers for support. One can also find a mentor or senior colleague who has been through the stresses and strains of practice for decades and from whom one can benefit. Physicians can ask a mentor to dinner periodically and try to share some of one's struggles with an older, wiser physician. It is also helpful to use consultants for difficult cases so one is not required to figure out every problem on one's own.

Perhaps one of the best ways to prevent a growing dependence on substances to alter one's mental state is to retain the services of a personal physician early in one's career. If all physicians could commit to the idea that they will not prescribe for themselves, this practice would go a long way to prevent addictive problems in physicians. Relying on another physician's judgment about one's treatment needs appears to be obvious, but it goes against the grain of the independent and rugged individualist ethos of medicine. Physicians tend to fear dependency, so they react by becoming counterdependent and not needing anyone to help them.

The problem of chemical dependency in physicians cannot be solved simply by self-monitoring. A certain subgroup of physicians who may be genetically predisposed to the use of chemical alteration of their physiology will probably drift in that direction, no matter what preventive efforts are instituted. However, all physicians have a responsibility to colleagues as well as to themselves. It is imperative for all physicians to be educated about reporting laws in their state or province and to recognize this responsibility for monitoring the profession themselves (Farber et al. 2005). If physicians fail to provide oversight on one another, other governmental bodies will take over for them.

Even before impairment to practice is in evidence, physicians may note that colleagues are drinking too much or prescribing for themselves in a way that is bound to lead to difficulty. Sometimes when one or two colleagues sit down with a physician and express their concern, it can serve as a wake-up call for that physician about the ways that others are viewing him or her. Some physicians may act defensively, but at least the seed has been planted for them to reflect more about their coping with stress.

One of the most fundamental ways to prevent problems in the life of a physician is to access mental healthcare when necessary. The resistance to seeking help from a psychiatrist, psychologist, or other mental health professional is pervasive throughout the life cycle of a physician. In a study of medical students, only 22% of those who had screened positive for depression actually used mental health services (Givens and Tija 2002). In the subsample of depressed students who contemplated suicide, only 42% received treatment.

The prevention of professional boundary violations requires a special kind of self-monitoring because what happens between the physician and patient generally occurs in the privacy of an office where confidentiality may be extremely important. One can use the professional boundaries identified in Chapter 7 ("Professional Boundary Violations") as a way of developing a mental checklist of how one relates to each patient. Questions that physicians can ask themselves include

- Am I spending more time with this patient than I really need to?
- Am I sexually attracted to this patient?
- Am I wanting to give special treatment to this patient?
- Am I slowly developing a dual relationship in which I am exploiting this patient's dependency and vulnerability?

Perhaps the most important question that can be asked in the context of preventing boundary violations is this: Is there anything I'm doing with this patient that I could not mention to a colleague or consultant? A corollary is whether there is anything that is being left out of the medical record because it would be embarrassing to include. In this manner, physicians are responding to the community standard of practice by noting whether their behavior is in some way at odds with those standards. Obviously, physicians should also use consultants when they get into these situations so they have someone else who can be objective to guide them on how to handle complicated patients. The fundamental principle is that anything one is doing with a patient should be part of a thoughtfully designed treatment plan.

Preventive Measures for Marriages, Partnerships, and Personal Relationships

One's spouse or partner is often taken for granted by physicians. They figure that they can count on this individual's love, so if they work too much or fret too often, they need not worry that they will lose the most important relationship. This type of thinking leads to the psychology of postponement noted in Chapter 1. The marriage or partnership will take care of itself, so it can wait until other things are addressed first.

The lack of attention to one's most personal relationships is one of the central problems that physicians face. It is ironic that the spouse or partner is potentially the most important source of support but also the first casualty of overwork and the stress of medical practice (Gabbard and Menninger 1988).

One simple preventive measure that can easily be implemented is a routine practice of speaking to one another each evening (Myers 2001). No matter how tired or distracted one is at the end of the day, time should be made for chatting about each partner's day in some detail so there is a sense of ongoing continuity in the couple's lives. In the study of physicians and spouses noted in Chapter 10, the 43 physicians in the study who had never considered or sought marital counseling were compared with 91 physicians who had. The physicians who sought marital counseling averaged 30.5 minutes per day talking with their spouses, whereas those who neither considered nor sought marital counseling averaged 57.3 minutes per day talking (Gabbard et al. 1987). Although cause and effect cannot clearly be established in these findings, they are certainly consistent with the idea that couples who communicate may have less need for marital counseling.

Other preventive measures apply to all couples. Needs must be made explicit to one another so there is no expectation of mind-reading. Responsibilities must be shared between the partners or spouses. Ultimately, neither partner can obtain everything that he or she wants, so compromise and concession are critically important. Each partner must be willing to give and take and to meet each other halfway. There is no magic in finding the perfect solution.

One important topic for communication is shared responsibilities for household work and children. Often, assumptions are made without clear negotiation about the division of labor. Physicians often work long hours because they are convinced that they are indispensable. Physicians may feel that they cannot hand a patient over to a partner or to someone else who is covering for them because only they can treat the patient in exactly the right way. Hence delegation becomes a last resort for many physicians. As noted in Chapter 1, those who cannot delegate consign themselves to overwork. Intimately related to the feeling of indispensability is the secret fantasy of omnipotence. Physicians may feel that if they invest the time and effort, any problem can be solved. If they are anything less than 100% committed, they feel they are depriving the patient of their knowledge and skill. As noted in Chapter 10, an important function of the spouse or partner is to say to the physician, "You really aren't as great as your patients think you are."

A sexual relationship is often relegated to a sometime thing because each partner is exhausted. Hence time for sexual relations must be built into the busy schedule of the physician because avoidance of sexuality can easily become a chronic pattern.

A sound practice for all marriages is to find something that the couple can do together—a hobby, an activity, or simply a date to dinner or a movie. If there is some sense of common enjoyment and pleasure in a nonmedical pursuit, the relationship takes on greater breadth and depth and is more likely to withstand stressors that threaten it.

Finally, the marriage or partnership depends not only on communication but also on listening. One of the best prophylactic measures is for each partner to listen to the other without judgment or distraction. Even if one partner disagrees with the other, a sense of listening, empathically validating the other's point of view, and respecting that perspective strengthens the relationship. Each partner has a legitimate perspective, however different from the other. Hence making a sincere effort at mentalizing what the other person is experiencing and feeling results in a feeling of being valued and "heard." Physicians tend to be controlling, and they must be wary of trying to make their spouse or partner think exactly the way they do.

Key Points

- Prevention is complicated, multifaceted, and never wholly successful.
- Selection of medical students must take into account virtues other than cognitive skills.
- Longitudinal studies demonstrate that professionalism problems in medical school may be linked to further disciplinary actions by state and provincial licensing boards.
- Much of professionalism teaching occurs informally in the so-called hidden curriculum.
- Long hours at work alone are not responsible for burnout. Seeking peer support and balancing work and family may help avoid burnout.
- The practice of self-monitoring must begin early so that physicians can note the first indications of difficulties.
- Daily communication with one's spouse or partner is a solid preventive practice that all physicians should consider.

Appendix

Resources and Web Sites

Federation of State Physician Health Programs (www.fsphp.org)   This site lists all of the states that have physician health programs and how to access what those programs have to offer.

Canadian Medical Association Centre for Physician Health and Well-Being (1-877-CMA-4-YOU [1-877-262-4968]; www.cma.ca)   This site has a link to the Canadian Physician Health Network and each provincial/territorial physician support program in Canada.

American Foundation for Suicide Prevention (www.afsp.org)   This site explains the foundation's physician depression and suicide prevention project. The project includes a film on physician depression and suicide and outreach to medical students, residents, and physicians at risk for suicide.

Physician Litigation Stress Resource Center (www.physicianlitigationstress.org) This site provides physicians and other health care professionals with the resources they need to understand and cope with the personal and professional stress created by involvement in a medical malpractice case or an adverse outcome that may result in litigation.

American Academy on Communication in Healthcare (www.aachonline.org) This site is a resource for physicians to improve their communication with patients.

The Journal of Humane Medicine and the Medical Humanities. Cell 2 Soul (www.cell2soul.org)   This e-publication is free and dedicated to exploring the humanities in patient care, thought, and experience.

Center for Personalized Education for Physicians (www.cpepdoc.org)   This site is a resource for physician evaluation, assessment, and education in an objective and neutral environment. It is nonpunitive and nonadversarial.

References

Adams D: Recovering physicians beating the odds. Am Med News 44 (December 24/31): 48, 2001

Albanese M, Snow MH, Skochelak SE, et al: Assessing personal qualities in medical school admissions. Acad Med 78:313–321, 2003

Allen J, Columbus M: Assessing Alcohol Problems: A Guide for Clinicians and Researchers. Rockville, MD, National Institute on Alcohol Abuse and Alcoholism, 1995

Allen J, Litten R, Fertig J: A review of research on the Alcohol Use Disorders Identification Test (AUDIT). Alcohol Clin Exp Res 21:613–619, 1997

American Foundation for Suicide Prevention: Physician Depression and Suicide Prevention Project, 2002. Information available at: http://www.afsp.org.

American Medical Association Council on Ethical and Judicial Affairs: Sexual misconduct in the practice of medicine. JAMA 266:2741–2745, 1991

American Psychiatric Association: Appendix I: outline for cultural formulation and glossary of culture-bound syndromes, in Diagnostic and Statistical Manual of Mental Disorders, 4th Edition, Text Revision. Washington, DC, American Psychiatric Association, 2000a

American Psychiatric Association: Diagnostic and Statistical Manual of Mental Disorders, 4th Edition, Text Revision. Washington, DC, American Psychiatric Association, 2000b

American Psychiatric Association: Practice Guidelines for the Treatment of Psychiatric Disorders: Assessment and Treatment of Patients With Suicidal Behaviors, Compendium 2004. Washington, DC, American Psychiatric Association, 2004, pp 835–1027

Anderson LP: Acculturative stress: a theory of relevance to Black Americans. Clin Psychol Rev 11:685–702, 1991

Andrews LW: Substance-impaired physicians: treating doctors and protecting patients. Journal of Medical Licensure and Discipline 91:7–12, 2005

Anthony JC, Chen CY: Epidemiology of drug dependence, in The American Psychiatric Publishing Textbook of Substance Abuse Treatment, 3rd Edition. Edited by Galanter M, Kleber HD. Washington, DC, American Psychiatric Publishing, 2004, pp 55–72

Arnold L, Stern DT: What is medical professionalism?, in Measuring Medical Professionalism. Edited by Stern DT. New York, Oxford University Press, 2006, pp 15–38

Associated Press: Child Heart Surgeon Drummond-Webb Dies. Little Rock, Arkansas. Sunday, December 26, 2004, 6:54 P.M.

Atkinson RM: Age-specific treatment programs for older adult alcoholics, in Alcohol Use Among U.S. Minorities. Edited by Gomberg ESL, Hegedus AM, Zucker RA. Rockville, MD, National Institute on Alcohol Abuse and Alcoholism, 1998, pp 425–435

Baldwin PJ, Dodd M, Wrate RW: Young doctors' health, I: how do working conditions affect attitudes, health, and performance? Journal of Social Science and Medicine 45:35–40, 1997

Basco MR: Never Good Enough. New York, Free Press, 1999

Bateman A, Fonagy P: Effectiveness of partial hospitalization in the treatment of border-line personality disorder: a randomized controlled trial. Am J Psychiatry 156:1563–1569, 1999

Bateman A, Fonagy P: Treatment of borderline personality disorder with psychoanalytically oriented partial hospitalization: an 18-month follow-up. Am J Psychiatry 158:36–42, 2001

Bateman A, Fonagy P: Mentalization-Based Treatment: A Practical Guide. New York, Oxford University Press, 2006

Bauman KA: Physician suicide. Arch Fam Med 4:672–673, 1995

Baxter EA: The turn of the tide. Psychiatr Serv 49:1297–1298, 1998

Beck AT, Freeman A: Cognitive Therapy of Personality Disorders. New York, Guilford, 1990

Beck AT, Rush AJ, Shaw BF, et al: Cognitive Therapy of Depression. New York, Guilford, 1979

Beevers CG, Miller IW: Perfectionism, cognitive bias, and hopelessness as prospective predictors of suicidal ideation. Suicide Life Threat Behav 34:126–137, 2004

Bergman SJ, Surrey JL: Couple therapy: a relational approach, in The Complexity of Connection: Writings from the Stone Center's Jean Baker Miller Training Institute. Edited by Jordan JV, Walker M, Hartling LM. New York, Guilford, 2004, pp 167–193

Berkowitz RI: Behavior therapies, in The American Psychiatric Publishing Textbook of Clinical Psychiatry, 4th Edition. Edited by Hales RE, Yudofsky SC. Washington, DC, American Psychiatric Publishing, 2003, pp 1225–1244

Berwick DM, Leape LL: Perfect is possible. Newsweek, Oct 16, 2006, pp 70–71

Bloom JD, Nadelson CC, Notman MT (eds): Physician Sexual Misconduct. Washington, DC, American Psychiatric Press, 1999

Book HE: How to Practice Brief Psychodynamic Psychotherapy: A Core Conflictual Relationship Theme Method. Washington, DC, American Psychological Association, 1998

Bradford JM: The neurobiology, neuropharmacology and pharmacological treatment of the paraphilias and compulsive sexual behavior. Can J Psychiatry 46:26–34, 2001

Brody J: Hidden plague of alcohol abuse by the elderly. New York Times, April 2, 2002, p F7

Brogan DJ, Frank E, Elon L, et al: Harassment of lesbians as medical students and physicians. JAMA 282:1290, 1292, 1999

Brotherton S, Simon F, Etzel S: U.S. graduate medical education, 2001–2002. JAMA 288:1073–1078, 2002

Brotherton SE, Rockey PH, Etzel SI: U.S. graduate medical education, 2004–2005. JAMA 294:1075–1082, 2005

Browne A, Finkelhor D: Impact of child sexual abuse: a review of the research. Psychol Bull 99:66–77, 1986

Burns DD: Feeling Good: The New Mood Therapy Revised and Updated. New York, William Morrow, 1999

Campbell FR: Aftermath of suicide: the clinician's role, in American Psychiatric Publishing Textbook of Suicide Assessment and Management. Edited by Simon RI, Hales RE. Washington, DC, American Psychiatric Publishing, 2006, pp 459–476

Canive JM, Castillo DT, Tuason VB: The Hispanic veteran, in Culture and Psychotherapy: A Guide to Clinical Practice. Edited by Tseng W-S, Streltzer J. Washington, DC, American Psychiatric Publishing, 2001, pp 157–172

Carpenter LM, Swerdlow AJ, Fear NT: Mortality of doctors in different specialties: findings from a cohort of 20,000 NHS consultants. Occup Environ Med 54:388–395, 1997

Carroll KM, Ball SA, Martino S: Cognitive, behavioral and motivational therapies, in The American Psychiatric Publishing Textbook of Substance Abuse Treatment, 3rd Edition. Edited by Galanter M, Kleber HD. Washington, DC, American Psychiatric Publishing, 2004, pp 365–376

Carter JH: Impaired black physicians: a methodology for detection and rehabilitation. J Nat Med Assoc 81:663–667, 1989

Caspi A, McClay J, Moffitt TE, et al: Role of genotype in the cycle of violence in maltreated children. J Sci 297:851–854, 2002

Celenza A: Sexual Boundary Violations: Therapeutic, Supervisory, and Academic Contexts. Lanham, MD, Jason Aronson, 2007

Celenza A, Gabbard GO: Analysts who commit sexual boundary violations: a lost cause? J Am Psychoanal Assoc 51:618–636, 2003

Center C, Davis M, Detre T, et al: Confronting depression and suicide in physicians: a consensus statement. JAMA 289:3161–3166, 2003

Chemtob CM, Hamada RS, Bauer G, et al: Patients' suicides: frequency and impact on psychiatrists. Am J Psychiatry 145:224–228, 1988

Chren MM, Landefeld CS, Murray TH: Doctors, drug companies, and gifts. JAMA 262:3448–3451, 1989

Clarkin JR, Levy KN, Lenzenweger MF, et al: Evaluating three treatments for borderline personality disorder: a multiwave study. Am J Psychiatry 164:922–928, 2007

Cloninger CR: Genetics of substance abuse, in The American Psychiatric Publishing Textbook of Substance Abuse Treatment, 3rd Edition. Edited by Galanter M, Kleber HD. Washington, DC, American Psychiatric Publishing, 2004, pp 73–79

Coccaro EF, Kavoussi RJ: Fluoxetine and impulsive aggressive behavior in personality-disordered subjects. Arch Gen Psychiatry 54:1081–1088, 1997

Comas-Diaz L, Jacobsen FM: Ethnocultural transference and countertransference in the therapeutic dyad. Am J Orthopsychiatry 61:392–402, 1991

Coombs RH: The medical marriage, in Psychological Aspects of Medical Training. Edited by Coombs RH, Vincent CE. Springfield, IL, Charles C Thomas, 1971

Coombs RH: Drug-Impaired Professionals. Cambridge, MA, Harvard University Press, 1997

Crits-Christoph P, McCalmont E, Weiss RD, et al: Impact of psychosocial treatments on associated problems of cocaine-dependent patients. J Consult Clin Psychol 69:825–830, 2001

Croasdale M: Women found more likely to burn out from practice stress. Am Med News 48:1–2, 2005

Dehlendorf CE, Wolfe SM: Physicians disciplined for sex-related offenses. JAMA 279:1883–1888, 1998

Delis D, Kramer JH, Kaplan E, et al: California Verbal Learning Test, 2nd Edition. San Antonio, TX, Psychological Corporation, 2000

Derdeyn AP: The physician's work and marriage. Int J Psychiatry Med 9:297–306, 1978

Dickstein LJ: Health Awareness Workshop Reference Manual. Louisville, KY, Proactive Press, 1998

Dilts SJ, Gendel MH: Substance use disorders, in The Handbook of Physician Health. Edited by Goldman LS, Myers M, Dickstein LJ. Chicago, IL, American Medical Association, 2000, pp 118–137

Doherty WJ, Burge SK: Divorce among physicians: comparisons with other occupational groups. JAMA 261:2374–2377, 1989

Domino KB, Hornbein TF, Polissar NL, et al: Risk factors for relapse in health care professionals with substance use disorders. JAMA 293:1453–1460, 2005

Donohoe M: Urine trouble: practical, legal and ethical issues surrounding mandated drug testing of physicians. J Clin Ethics 16:85–96, 2005

Dorsey ER, Jarjoura D, Rutecki GW: The influence of controllable lifestyle and sex on the specialty choices of graduating U.S. medical students, 1996–2003. Acad Med 80:791–796, 2005

Du N: Asian American patients, in Clinical Manual of Cultural Psychiatry. Edited by Lim RF. Washington, DC, American Psychiatric Publishing, 2006, pp 69–117

Ellis JJ, Inbody DR: Psychotherapy with physicians' families: when attributes in medical practice become liabilities in family life. Am J Psychother 42:380–388, 1988

Epstein RS: Keeping the Boundaries. Washington, DC, American Psychiatric Press, 1994

Epstein RS, Simon RI: The exploitation index: an early warning indicator of boundary violations in psychotherapy. Bull Menninger Clin 54:450–465, 1990

Farber NJ, Gilibert SG, Aboff BM, et al: Physicians' willingness to report impaired colleagues. Soc Sci Med 61:1772–1775, 2005

Federation of State Medical Boards: A Guide to the Essentials of a Modern Medical Practice, 9th Edition, Section XI: Impaired Physician. Dallas, TX, Federation of State Medical Boards, 2000, p 26

Federation of State Medical Boards: Section I: introduction, in Addressing Sexual Boundaries: Guidelines for State Medical Boards, May 2006. Available at: http://www.fsmb.org/pdf/grpol_sexual boundaries.pdf. Accessed April 4, 2007.

Feinberg ME, Button TMM, Neiderhiser JM, et al: Parenting and adolescent antisocial behavior and depression: evidence of genotype x parenting environment interaction. Arch Gen Psychiatry 64:457–465, 2007

Fine C: Married to Medicine: An Intimate Portrait of Doctors' Wives. New York, Atheneum, 1981

Fine C: No Time to Say Goodbye: Surviving the Suicide of a Loved One. New York, Doubleday, 1997

Fletcher RH, Fletcher SW: Here come the couples. Ann Intern Med 119:628–630, 1993

Flett GL, Hewitt PL (eds): Perfectionism: Theory, Research, and Treatment. Washington, DC, American Psychological Association, 2002

Fonagy P, Target M: Attachment Theory and Psychoanalysis. New York, Other Press, 2001

Fong TW: Understanding and managing compulsive sexual behaviors. Psychiatry 3:51–58, 2006

Ford DE, Mead LA, Change PP, et al: Depression is a risk factor in coronary artery disease in men: the precursors study. Arch Intern Med 158:1422–1426, 1998

Forney P, Forney M, Fischer P, et al: Sociocultural correlates of substance use among medical students. J Drug Educ 18:97–108, 1988

Frank E, Dingle AD: Self-reported depression and suicide attempts among U.S. women physicians. Am J Psychiatry 156:1887–1894, 1999

Frank E, Brogan DJ, Mokdad AH, et al: Health-related behaviors of women physicians vs other women in the United States. Arch Intern Med158:342–348, 1998

Frank E, Biola H, Burnett CA: Mortality rates and causes among U.S. physicians. Am J Prev Med 19:155–159, 2000

Frick DE: Nonsexual boundary violations in psychiatric treatment, in American Psychiatric Press Review of Psychiatry, Vol 13. Edited by Oldham JM, Riba MB. Washington, DC, American Psychiatric Press, 1994, pp 415–432

Gabbard GO: The role of compulsiveness in the normal physician. JAMA 254:2926–2929, 1985

Gabbard GO: Sexual misconduct, in American Psychiatric Press Review of Psychiatry, Vol 13. Edited by Oldham JM, Riba MB. Washington, DC, American Psychiatric Press, 1994, pp 433–456

Gabbard GO: Countertransference: the emerging common ground. Int J Psychoanal 76:475–485, 1995a

Gabbard GO: Transference and countertransference in the psychotherapy of therapists charged with sexual misconduct. Psychiatr Ann 25:100–105, 1995b

Gabbard GO: Long-Term Psychodynamic Psychotherapy. Washington, DC, American Psychiatric Publishing, 2004

Gabbard GO: Mind, brain, and personality disorders. Am J Psychiatry 162:648–655, 2005a

Gabbard GO: Psychodynamic Psychiatry in Clinical Practice, 4th Edition. Washington, DC, American Psychiatric Publishing, 2005b

Gabbard GO, Allison SE: Psychodynamic treatment, in The American Psychiatric Publishing Textbook of Suicide Assessment and Management. Edited by Simon RI, Hales RE. Washington, DC, American Psychiatric Publishing, 2006, pp 221–234

Gabbard GO, Lester EP: Boundaries and Boundary Violations in Psychoanalysis. Washington DC, American Psychiatric Publishing, 2003

Gabbard GO, Martinez M: Professional boundary violations by physicians. Journal of Medical Licensure and Discipline 91:10–15, 2005

Gabbard GO, Menninger RW (eds): Medical Marriages. Washington, DC, American Psychiatric Press, 1988

Gabbard GO, Menninger RW: The psychology of postponement in the medical marriage. JAMA 262:2378–2381, 1989

Gabbard GO, Nadelson CC: Professional boundaries in the physician-patient relationship. JAMA 273:1445–1449, 1995

Gabbard GO, Menninger RW, Coyne L: Sources of conflict in the medical marriage. Am J Psychiatry 144:567–572, 1987

Gartrell NK, Milliken N, Goodson WH, et al: Physician-patient sexual contact: prevalence and problems. West J Med 157:139–143, 1992

Garvey M, Tuason VB: Physician marriages. J Clin Psychiatry 40:129–131, 1979

Gastfriend DR: Physician substance abuse and recovery: what does it mean for physicians—and everyone else? JAMA 293:1513–1515, 2005

Gay and Lesbian Medical Association: Guidelines for Care of Lesbian, Gay, Bisexual, and Transgender Patients. November 1, 2006. Available at: www.glma.org.

Gelfand DV, Podnos YD, Carmichael JC, et al: Effect of the 80-hour work week in resident burnout. Arch Surg 139:933–938, 2004

Gendel MH: Treatment adherence in physicians. Prim Psychiatry 12:48–54, 2005

Gendel MH: Substance misuse and substance-related disorders in forensic psychiatry. Psychiatr Clin North Am 29:649–673, 2006

Gerber LA: Married to Their Careers: Career and Family Dilemmas in Doctors' Lives. New York, Tavistock, 1983

Giesen-Bloo J, van Dyck R, Spinhoven P, et al: Outpatient psychotherapy for borderline personality disorder: randomized trial of schema-focused therapy vs. transference-focused psychotherapy. Arch Gen Psychiatry 63:649–658, 2006

Gilligan C: In a Different Voice. Cambridge, MA, Harvard University Press, 1982

Gitlin M: A psychiatrist's reaction to a patient's suicide. Am J Psychiatry 156:1630–1634, 1999

Gitlin M: Psychiatrist reactions to patient suicide, in Textbook of Suicide Assessment and Management. Edited by Simon RI, Hales RE. Washington, DC, American Psychiatric Publishing, 2006, pp 477–494

Givens JL, Tija J: Depressed medical students use of mental health services and barriers to use. Acad Med 77:918–921, 2002

Glick ID, Borus JF: Marital and family therapy for troubled physicians and their families: a bridge over troubled waters. JAMA 251:1855–1858, 1984

Glymour MM, Saha S, Bigby JA: Physician race and ethnicity, professional satisfaction, and work-related stress: results from the physician worklife study. J Nat Med Assoc 96:1283–1294, 2004

Gold LH, Metzner JL: Psychiatric employment evaluations and the Health Insurance Portability and Accountability Act. Am J Psychiatry 163:1878–1882, 2006

Gold MS, Frost-Pineda K: Letter to the editor. Ann Intern Med 144:861, 2006

Gold MS, Byars JA, Frost-Pineda K: Occupational exposure and addictions for physicians: case studies and theoretical implications. Psychiatr Clin North Am 27:745–753, 2004

Gold MS, Melker RJ, Dennis DM, et al: Fentanyl abuse and dependence: further evidence for second hand exposure hypothesis. J Addict Dis 25:15–21, 2006

Goldberg M: Conjoint therapy of male physicians and their wives. Psychiatr Opin 12:19–23, 1975

Golden CJ: Stroop Color and Word Test. Chicago, IL, Stoelting, 1976

Gonzalez CA, Griffith EEH, Ruiz P: Cross-cultural issues in psychiatric treatment, in Treatments of Psychiatric Disorders. Edited by Gabbard GO. Washington, DC, American Psychiatric Publishing, 2001, pp 47–67

Grant JE, Potenza MN, Hollander E, et al: Multicenter investigation of the opioid antagonist nalmefene in the treatment of pathological gambling. Am J Psychiatry 163:303–312, 2006

Greenberger D, Padesky CA: Mind Over Mood. New York, Guilford, 1995

Greenfield SF, Hennessy G: Assessment of the patient, in The American Psychiatric Publishing Textbook of Substance Abuse Treatment, 3rd Edition. Edited by Galanter M, Kleber HD. Washington, DC, American Psychiatric Publishing, 2004, pp 101–119

Griffith EEH: Personal narrative and an African-American perspective on medical ethics. J Am Acad Psychiatry Law 33:371–381, 2005

Group for the Advancement of Psychiatry, Committee on Cultural Psychiatry: Cultural Assessment in Clinical Psychiatry. Washington, DC, American Psychiatric Publishing, 2002

Gunderson DC: Women in medicine. Colorado Physician Health Program News 5:2, 11–13, 2006

Gunderson JG, Gabbard GO: Making the case for psychoanalytic therapies in the current psychiatric environment. J Am Psychoanal Assoc 47:679–704, 1999

Gutheil TG, Gabbard GO: The concept of boundaries in clinical practice: theoretical and risk-management dimensions. Am J Psychiatry 150:188–196, 1993

Hamilton TK, Schweitzer RD: The cost of being perfect: perfectionism and suicide ideation in university students. Aust NZ J Psychiatry 34:829–835, 2000

Hawton K, Clements A, Simkin S, et al: Doctors who kill themselves: a study of the methods used for suicide. Q J Med 93:351–357, 2000

Hawton K, Clements A, Sakarovitch C, et al: Suicide in doctors: a study of risk according to gender, seniority and specialty in medical practitioners in England and Wales, 1979–1995. J Epidemiol Community Health 55:296–300, 2001

Hendin H, Lipschitz A, Maltsberger JT, et al: Therapists' reactions to patients' suicides. Am J Psychiatry 157:2022–2027, 2000

Hendrie HC, Clair DK, Brittain HM, et al: A study of anxiety/depressive symptoms of medical students, house staff, and their spouses/partners. J Nerv Ment Dis 178:204–207, 1990

Hilsenroth MJ: A programmatic study of short-term psychodynamic psychotherapy: assessment, process, outcome, and training. Psychother Res 17:31–45, 2007

Hojat M, Gonnella JS, Mangione S, et al: Empathy in medical students as related to academic performance, clinical competence, and gender. Med Educ 36:522–527, 2002

Holmes VF, Rich CL: Suicide among physicians, in Suicide Over the Life Cycle: Risk Factors, Assessment and Treatment of Suicidal Patients. Edited by Blumenthal S, Kupfer D. Washington, DC, American Psychiatric Press, 1990, pp 599–615

Hooper HE: The Hooper Visual Organization Test. Beverly Hills, CA, Western Psychological Services, 1958

Horvath AO: The therapeutic relationship: research and theory. Psychother Res 15:3–7, 2005

Hsu K, Marshall V: Prevalence of depression and distress in a large sample of Canadian residents, interns, and fellows. Am J Psychiatry 144:1561–1566, 1987

Hughes PH, Brandenburg N, Baldwin DC, et al: Prevalence of substance use among U.S. physicians. JAMA 267:2333–2339, 1992

Jamison KR: Night Falls Fast: Understanding Suicide. New York, Knopf, 1999, p 268

Jamison KR: Foreword, in Touched by Suicide: Hope and Healing After Loss. Edited by Myers MF, Fine C. New York, Gotham/Penguin Books, 2006, p xiii

Johnson SH: Judicial review of disciplinary action for sexual misconduct in the practice of medicine. JAMA 270:1596–1600, 1993

Jones SA, Gabbard GO: Marital therapy of physician couples, in Medical Marriages. Edited by Gabbard GO, Menninger RW. Washington, DC, American Psychiatric Press, 1988, pp 137–151

Kendler KS: Toward a philosophical structure for psychiatry. Am J Psychiatry 162:433–440, 2005

Kernberg OF: Severe Personality Disorders: Psychotherapeutic Strategies. New Haven, CT, Yale University Press, 1984

Khadivi A, Wetzler S, Wilson A: Manic indices on the Rorschach. J Pers Assess 69:365–375, 1997

Knight JR: A 35-year-old physician with opioid dependence. JAMA 292:1351–1357, 2004

Knight JR, Sanchez LT, Sherritt L, et al: Monitoring physician drug problems: attitudes of participants. J Addict Dis 21:27–36, 2002

Krakowski AJ: Stress and the practice of medicine, II: stressors, stresses and strains. Psychother Psychosom 38:11–23, 1982

Kramer M: Educational challenges of International Medical Graduates in psychiatric residencies. J Am Acad Psychoanal Dyn Psychiatry 34:163–171, 2006

Krell R, Miles J: Marital therapy of couples in which the husband is a physician. Am J Psychotherapy 30:267–275, 1976

Lambert EM, Holmboe ES: The relationship between specialty choice and gender of U.S. medical students, 1990–2003. Acad Med 80:797–802, 2005

Landrigan CP, Barger LK, Cade BE, et al: Interns' compliance with Accreditation Council for Graduate Medical Education. JAMA 296:1063–1070, 2006

Laws DR, Hudson SM, Ward T: The original model of relapse prevention with sex offenders, in Remaking Relapse Prevention with Sex Offenders: A Sourcebook. Edited
  by Laws DR, Hudson SM, Ward T. Thousand Oaks, CA, Sage, 2000, pp 3–26

Leape LL, Fromson JA: Problem doctors: is there a system-level solution? Ann Intern
  Med 144:107–115, 2006

Leichsenring F: Efficacy, indications, and applications of psychodynamic psychotherapy to
  specific disorders, in The American Psychiatric Publishing Textbook of Psychotherapeutic Treatments in Psychiatry. Edited by Gabbard GO. Washington, DC, American
  Psychiatric Publishing (in press)

Leichsenring F, Rabung S, Leibing E: The efficacy of short-term psychodynamic psychotherapy in specific psychiatric disorders: a meta-analysis. Arch Gen Psychiatry 61:1208–
  1216, 2004

Lim RF: Clinical Manual of Cultural Psychiatry. Washington, DC, American Psychiatric
  Publishing, 2006

Linehan MM: Cognitive-Behavioral Treatment of Borderline Personality Disorder. New
  York, Guilford, 1993a

Linehan MM: Skills Training Manual for Treating Borderline Personality Disorder. New
  York, Guilford, 1993b

Luborsky L: Principles of Psychoanalytic Psychotherapy: A Manual for Supportive-
  Expressive Treatment. New York, Basic Books, 1984

Mack AH, Lightdale HA: Substance-related disorders, in The American Psychiatric Publishing Textbook of Suicide Assessment and Management. Edited by Simon RI,
  Hales RE. Washington, DC, American Psychiatric Publishing, 2006, pp 347–364

Maltsberger JT: Treating the suicidal patient: basic principles. Ann NY Acad Sci 932:158–
  168, 2001

Maltsberger JT: Outpatient treatment, in The American Psychiatric Publishing Textbook
  of Suicide Assessment and Management. Edited by Simon RI, Hales RE. Washington, DC, American Psychiatric Publishing, 2006, pp 367–380

Mandell H, Spiro H: When Doctors Get Sick. New York, Plenum, 1987, p xi

Mann JJ, Waternaux C, Haas GL, et al: Toward a clinical model of suicidal behavior in
  psychiatric patients. Am J Psychiatry 156:181–189, 1999

Mansky PA: Issues in the recovery of physicians from addictive illnesses. Psychiatr Q
  70:107–122, 1999

Mansky PA: Impaired physicians, in The American Psychiatric Publishing Textbook of
  Substance Abuse Treatment, 3rd Edition. Edited by Galanter M, Kleber HD. Washington, DC, American Psychiatric Publishing, 2004, pp 575–583

Markovitz P: Pharmacotherapy of impulsivity, aggression, and related disorders, in Impulsivity and Aggression. Edited by Hollander E, Stein DJ, Zohar J. New York, Wiley,
  1995, pp 263–287

Marlatt GA, Gordon J (eds): Relapse Prevention: Maintenance Strategies in the Treatment
  of Addictive Behaviors. New York, Guilford, 1985

Mayfield D, McLeod G, Hall P: The CAGE questionnaire: validation of a new alcoholism
  screening instrument. Am J Psychiatry 131:1121–1123, 1974

McCann IL, Pearlman LA: Vicarious traumatization: a framework for understanding
  the psychological effects of working with victims. J Trauma Stress 3:131–149,
  1990

McCullough LB, Chervenak FA, Coverdale JH: Ethically justified guidelines for defining
  sexual boundaries between obstetrician-gynecologists and their patients. Am J Ob-
  stet Gynecol 175:496–500, 1996

McMurray JE, Linzer M, Konrad TR, et al: The work lives of women physicians: results from the physician work life study. The SGIM Career Satisfaction Study Group. J Gen Intern Med 15:372–380, 2000

McWilliams N: Psychoanalytic Psychotherapy: A Practitioner's Guide. New York, Guilford, 2004

Menninger KA: Psychological factors in the choice of medicine as a profession: part II. Bull Menninger Clin 21:99–106, 1957

Miles JE, Krell R, Lin T: The doctor's wife: mental illness and marital pattern. Int J Psychiatry Med 6:481–487, 1975

Miller JB, Stiver I: The Healing Connection. Boston, MA, Beacon Press, 1997

Miller WR, Rollnick S: Motivational Interviewing: Preparing People for Change, 2nd Edition. New York, Guilford, 2002

Moran M: Licensure language changed to avoid MH care stigma. Psychiatric News May 19, 2006, pp 23, 74

Morley L: Personality Assessment Inventory. Odessa, FL, Psychological Assessment Resources, 1991

Morrison J, Wickersham P: Physicians disciplined by a state medical board. JAMA 279:1889–1893, 1998

Mullan F: The metrics of the physician brain drain. N Engl J Med 353:1810–1818, 2005

Myers GE: Addressing the effects of culture on the boundary-keeping practices of psychiatry residents educated outside the United States. Acad Psychiatry 28:47–55, 2004

Myers MF: Overview: the female physician and her marriage. Am J Psychiatry 141:1386–1391, 1984

Myers MF: Doctors' Marriages: A Look at the Problems and Their Solutions, 2nd Edition. New York, Plenum, 1994

Myers MF: Cracks in the mirror: when a psychiatrist treats physicians and their families, in In a Perilous Calling: The Hazards of Psychotherapy Practice. Edited by Sussman MB. New York, Wiley, 1995, pp 169–170

Myers MF: Abuse of residents: it's time to take action. Can Med Assoc J 154:1705–1708, 1996a

Myers MF: Physicians Living With Depression (videotape). Washington, DC, American Psychiatric Publishing, 1996b

Myers MF: The psychiatrist's role in the management of impaired colleagues. Directions in Psychiatry 15:1–8, 1996c

Myers MF: Intimate Relationships in Medical School: How to Make Them Work. Thousand Oaks, CA, Sage, 2000

Myers MF: The well-being of physician relationships. West J Med 174:30–33, 2001

Myers MF: How's your marriage, doctor? Physicians' Money Digest, May 15, 2002

Myers MF: How's your marriage, doctor? (revised). Physicians' Money Digest, March 2004

Myers MF: How's your marriage doctor? Physician's Money Digest, December 2005, p 39

Myers MF: Physician suicides leave many victims in their wake. Winnipeg Free Press, October 1, 2006

Myers MF: When Physicians Commit Suicide: Reflections of Those They Leave Behind (videotape). Vancouver, BC, Media Services, St Paul's Hospital, 1998

Myers MF, Dickstein LJ: Psychiatrists living with a mental illness, in Syllabus and Proceedings Summary, American Psychiatric Association Annual Meeting. Washington, DC, American Psychiatric Association, 1999–2007

Myers MF, Fine C: Touched By Suicide: Hope and Healing After Loss. New York, Gotham/Penguin Books, 2006

Nadelson CC, Notman MT: The woman physician's marriage, in Medical Marriages. Edited by Gabbard GO, Menninger RW. Washington DC, American Psychiatric Press, 1988, pp 79–88

Nakajima GA, Chan YH, Lee K: Mental health issues for gay and lesbian Asian Americans, in Textbook of Homosexuality and Mental Health. Edited by Cabaj RP, Stein TS. Washington, DC, American Psychiatric Press, 1996, pp 563–581

Neser WB, Thomas J, Semenya K, et al: Obesity and hypertension in a longitudinal study of black physicians: the Meharry Cohort Study. J Chronic Dis 39:105–113, 1986

Nestler EJ: Is there a common molecular pathway for addiction? Nat Neurosci 8:1445–1449, 2005

Notman M, Nadelson C: Medicine: a career conflict for women. Am J Psychiatry 130:1123–1127, 1973

O'Reilly KB: Turning to peer support after medical errors. Am Med News 49:1–4, 2006

Okie S: An elusive balance: residents' work hours and the continuity of care. N Engl J Med 356:2665–2667, 2007

Papadakis MA, Teherani A, Banach MA, et al: Disciplinary action by medical boards and prior behavior in medical school. N Engl J Med 353:2673–2682, 2005

Pare M: Boundary lines: is disclosing your own mental illness the right thing to do? Medical Post, Toronto, ON, Nov 14, 2006, pp 56–57

Parsons OA, Farr SP: Neuropsychology of alcohol and drug use, in Handbook of Clinical Neuropsychology. Edited by Filskov S, Boll T. New York, Wiley Interscience, 1981, pp 320–365

Partington JE, Leiter RG: Partington's Pathway Test. Psychological Services Center Bulletin 1:9–20, 1979

Petersen-Crair P, Marangell L, Flack J, et al: An impaired physician with complex comorbidity. Am J Psychiatry 160:850–854, 2003

Post D, Weddington W: The impact of culture on physician stress and coping. J Nat Med Assoc 89:585–590, 1997

Primm AB: African American patients, in Clinical Manual of Cultural Psychiatry. Edited by Lim RF. Washington, DC, American Psychiatric Publishing, 2006, pp 35–68

Pyskoty CE, Richman JA, Faherty JA: Psychosocial aspects and mental health of minority medical students. Acad Med 65:581–585, 1990

Rabin D, Rabin PL, Rabin R: Occasional notes. Compounding the ordeal of ALS: isolation from my fellow physicians. N Engl J Med 307:506–509, 1982

Rao NR, Kramer M, Saunders R, et al: An annotated bibliography of professional literature on International Medical Graduates. Acad Psychiatry 31:68–83, 2007

Reiss D, Hetherington EM, Plomin R, et al: Genetic questions for environmental studies: differential parenting and psychopathology in adolescence. Arch Gen Psychiatry 52:925–936, 1995

Rhoades J: Overwork. JAMA 237:2615–2618, 1977

Richardson DA, Becker M, Frank RR, et al: Assessing medical students' perceptions of mistreatment in their second and third years. Acad Med 72:728–730, 1997

Rinne T, van den Brink W, Wouters L, et al: SSRI treatment of borderline personality disorder: a randomized placebo-controlled clinical trial for female patients with borderline personality disorder. Am J Psychiatry 159:2048–2054, 2002

Rollman BL, Mead LA, Wang NY, et al: Medical specialty and the incidence of divorce. N Engl J Med 336:800–803, 1997

Rose KD, Rosow I: Marital stability among physicians. Calif Med 16:95–99, 1972

Rotter J: Incomplete Sentences Test. New York, Psychological Corporation, 1950

Ryback RS: Naltrexone in the treatment of adolescent sexual offenders. J Clin Psychiatry 65:982–986, 2004

Salzman C, Wolfson AN, Schatzberg A, et al: Effect of fluoxetine on anger in symptomatic volunteers with borderline personality disorder. J Clin Psychopharmacol 15:23–29, 1995

Schernhammer ES, Colditz GA: Suicide rates among physicians: a quantitative and gender assessment (meta-analysis). Am J Psychiatry 161:2295–2302, 2004

Sensky T: Cognitive-behavior therapy for patients with physical illnesses, in Cognitive-Behavior Therapy. Edited by Wright JH. Review of Psychiatry Vol 23. Series editors: JM Oldham, MB Riba. Washington, DC, American Psychiatric Publishing, 2004, pp 83–121

Shneidman ES: Autopsy of a Suicidal Mind. New York, Oxford University Press, 2004

Silverman M: Physicians and suicide, in The Handbook of Physician Health: An Essential Guide to Understanding the Healthcare Needs of Physicians. Edited by Goldman LS, Myers M, Dickstein LJ. Chicago, IL, American Medical Association, 2000, pp 95–117

Simon RI: Patient safety versus freedom of movement: coping with uncertainty, in The American Psychiatric Publishing Textbook of Suicide Assessment and Management. Edited by Simon RI, Hales RE. Washington, DC, American Psychiatric Publishing, 2006

Skinner HA: The drug abuse screening test. Addict Behav 7:363–371, 1982

Skodol AE, Stout RL, McGlashan TH, et al: Co-occurrence of mood and personality disorders: a report from the Collaborative Longitudinal Personality Disorders Study (CLPS). Depress Anxiety 10:175–182, 1999

Smith MW: Ethnopsychopharmacology, in Clinical Manual of Cultural Psychiatry. Edited by Lim RF. Washington, DC, American Psychiatric Publishing, 2006, pp 207–235

Sobecks NW, Justice AC, Hinze S, et al: When doctors marry doctors: a survey exploring the professional and family lives of young physicians. Ann Intern Med 130:312–319, 1999

Sontag S: Illness As Metaphor. New York, Farrar, Straus, Giroux, 1978

Sotile WM, Sotile MO: The Medical Marriage: Sustaining Healthy Relationships for Physicians and Their Families. Chicago, IL, American Medical Association, 2000

Spickard A, Gabbe S, Christensen J: Mid-career burnout in generalist and specialist physicians. JAMA 288:1447–1450, 2002

Spreen O, Benton AL: Neurosensory Center Comprehensive Examination for Aphasia (NCCEA). Victoria, BC, Canada, University of Victoria Neuropsychology Laboratory, 1977

Steinbrook R: Imposing personal responsibility for health. N Engl J Med 355:753–756, 2006

Stern DT (ed): Measuring Medical Professionalism. New York, Oxford Press, 2006

Stern DT, Papadakis M: The developing physician: becoming a professional. N Engl J Med 355:1794–1799, 2006

Strasburger LH, Jorgenson L, Sutherland P: The prevention of psychotherapist sexual misconduct: avoiding the slippery slope. Am J Psychother 46:544–555, 1992

Svartberg M, Stiles TC, Seltzer MH: Randomized, controlled trial of the effectiveness of short-term dynamic psychotherapy and cognitive therapy for Cluster C personality disorders. Am J Psychiatry 161:810–817, 2004

Tamminga CA, Nestler EJ: Pathological gambling: focusing on the addiction, not the activity. Am J Psychiatry 163:180–181, 2006

Taragin MI, Wilczek AP, Karns ME, et al: Physician demographics and the risk of medical practice. Am J Med 93:537–542, 1992

Terman LM: Scientists and non-scientists in a group of 800 gifted men. Psychol Monogr 68:1–44, 1954

Thase ME: Cognitive-behavioral therapy for substance abuse, in American Psychiatric Press Review of Psychiatry, Vol 16. Edited by Dickstein LJ, Riba MB, Oldham JM. Washington, DC, American Psychiatric Press, 1997, pp 45–71

Thomas NK: Resident burnout. JAMA 292:2880–2889, 2004

Torre D, Wang NY, Mead LA, et al: Mortality in a prospective study of physicians. J Gen Intern Med 15(suppl):150, 2000

Vaillant GE, Sobowale NC, McArthur C: Some psychological vulnerabilities of physicians. N Engl J Med 287:372–375, 1972

van der Kolk BA: The compulsion to repeat the trauma: re-enactment, revictimization, and masochism. Psychiatr Clin North Am 12:389–411, 1989

Verghese A: Physicians and addiction. N Engl J Med 346:1510–1511, 2002

Verlander G: Female physicians: balancing career and family. Acad Psychiatry 28:331–336, 2004

Viswanathan R: Death anxiety, locus of control, and purpose in life of physicians: their relationship to patient death notification. Psychosomatics 37:339–345, 1996

Wagoner NE: Admission to medical school: selecting applicants with the potential for professionalism, in Measuring Medical Professionalism. Edited by Stern DT. New York, Oxford University Press, 2006, pp 235–264

Walzer RS: Impaired physicians: an overview and update of the legal issues. J Legal Med 11:131–198, 1990

Warhaft N: Alternative approaches to 12-Step attendance in the management of addicted physicians. Paper presented at the International Conference on Physician Health, Ottawa, ON, Canada, November 30–December 2, 2006

Wazana A, Primeau F: Ethical considerations in the relationship between physicians and the pharmaceutical industry. Psychiatr Clin North Am 25:647–663, 2002

Webb C: Taking care of myself, in Taking My Place in Medicine. Edited by Webb C. Thousand Oaks, CA, Sage, 2000, pp 97–118

Webb C, Smith S, Hawkins M, et al: Focus on African American medical students, in Taking My Place in Medicine. Edited by Webb C. Thousand Oaks, CA, Sage, 2000, pp 139–155

Wechsler D: The Wechsler Memory Scale, 3rd Edition. San Antonio, TX, Psychological Corporation, 1997

West CP, Huschka MM, Novotny PJ, et al: Association of perceived medical errors with resident distress and empathy: a prospective longitudinal study. JAMA 296:1071–1078, 2006

Wheeler JG, George WH, Stoner SA: Enhancing the relapse prevention model for sex offenders, in Relapse Prevention: Maintenance Strategies in the Treatment of Addictive Behaviors, 2nd Edition. Edited by Marlatt GA, Donovan DM. New York, Guilford, 2005, pp 333–362

Wilbers D, Veensstra G, van de Wiel HBM, et al: Sexual contact in the doctor-patient relationship in the Netherlands. Br Med J 304:1531–1534, 1992

Williams AP, Domnick-Pierre K, Vayda E, et al: Women in medicine: practice patterns and attitudes. Can Med Assoc J 143:194–201, 1990

Woodward CA, Williams AP, Ferrier B, et al: Time spent on professional activities and unwaged domestic work: is it different for male and female primary care workers who have children at home? Can Fam Physician 42:1928–1935, 1996

Wright JH: Computer-assisted cognitive-behavior therapy, in Cognitive-Behavior Therapy. Edited by Wright JH. Review of Psychiatry Vol 23. Series editors: JM Oldham, MB Riba. Washington, DC, American Psychiatric Publishing, 2004a, pp 55–82

Wright JH: Introduction, in Cognitive-Behavior Therapy. Edited by Wright JH. Review of Psychiatry Vol 23. Series editors: JM Oldham, MB Riba. Washington, DC, American Psychiatric Publishing, 2004b, pp xv–xxi

Wright JH, Basco MR: Getting Your Life Back: The Complete Guide to Recovery from Depression. New York, Free Press, 2001

Wright JH, Beck AT, Thase ME: Cognitive therapy, in The American Psychiatric Publishing Textbook of Clinical Psychiatry, 4th Edition. Edited by Hales RE, Yudofsky SC. Washington, DC, American Psychiatric Publishing, 2003, pp 1245–1284

Wright JH, Basco MR, Thase ME: Learning Cognitive-Behavior Therapy. Washington, DC, American Psychiatric Publishing, 2006, p ix

Index

*Page numbers printed in **boldface** type refer to tables or figures.*